The 30-DAY
ALZHEIMER'S SOLUTION

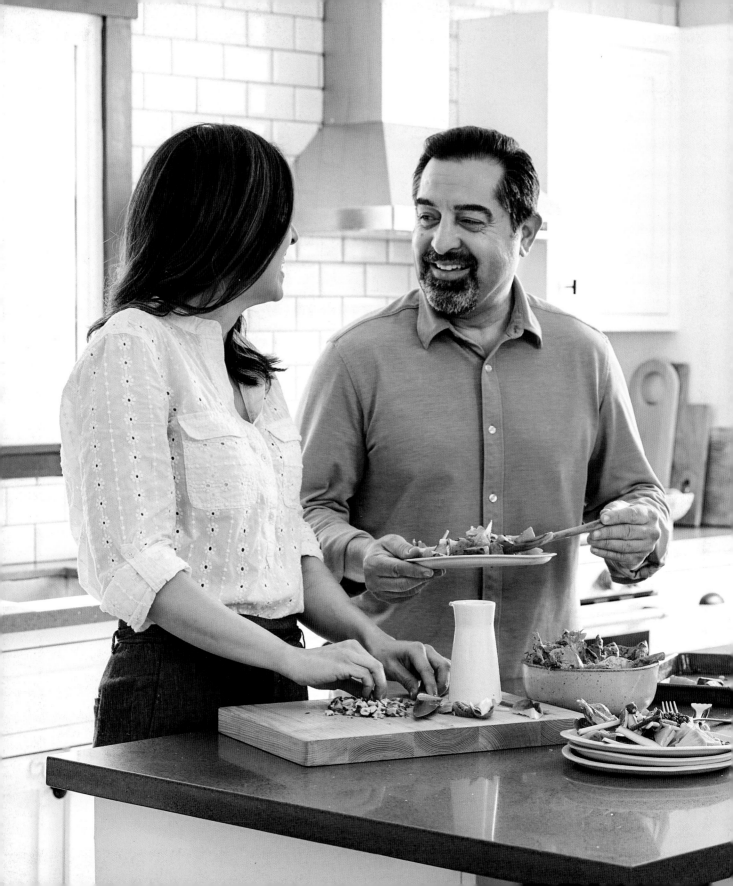

The 30-DAY
ALZHEIMER'S SOLUTION

THE DEFINITIVE FOOD AND LIFESTYLE GUIDE TO PREVENTING COGNITIVE DECLINE

Dean Sherzai *and* Ayesha Sherzai

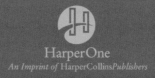

HarperOne
An Imprint of HarperCollins*Publishers*

ALSO BY DEAN AND AYESHA SHERZAI

The Alzheimer's Solution

THE 30-DAY ALZHEIMER'S SOLUTION. Copyright © 2021 by Dean Sherzai and Ayesha Sherzai. All rights reserved. Printed in Canada. No part of this book may be used or reproduced in any manner whatsoever without written permission except in the case of brief quotations embodied in critical articles and reviews. For information, address HarperCollins Publishers, 195 Broadway, New York, NY 10007.

HarperCollins books may be purchased for educational, business, or sales promotional use. For information, please email the Special Markets Department at SPsales@harpercollins.com.

FIRST EDITION

Interior and cover photographs by Colin Price Photography
Designed by Kris Tobiassen of Matchbook Digital

Library of Congress Cataloging-in-Publication Data

Names: Sherzai, Dean, author. | Sherzai, Ayesha, author.
Title: The 30-day Alzheimer's solution : the definitive food and lifestyle guide to preventing cognitive decline / Dean Sherzai, Ayesha Sherzai.
Other titles: Thirty-day Alzheimer's solution
Description: First edition. | San Francisco : HarperOne, [2021] | Includes bibliographical references and index.
Identifiers: LCCN 2020044115 (print) | LCCN 2020044116 (ebook) | ISBN 9780062996954 (hardcover) | ISBN 9780062996961 (ebook other) | ISBN 9780063068223 (ebook other) | ISBN 9780063068216 (ebook other)
Subjects: LCSH: Alzheimer's disease—Prevention—Popular works. | Alzheimer's disease—Diet therapy—Popular works. | Cooking—Popular works.
Classification: LCC RC523.2 .S5358 2021 (print) | LCC RC523.2 (ebook) | DDC 616.8/3110654—dc23
LC record available at https://lccn.loc.gov/2020044115
LC ebook record available at https://lccn.loc.gov/2020044116

21 22 23 24 25 TC 10 9 8 7 6 5 4 3 2

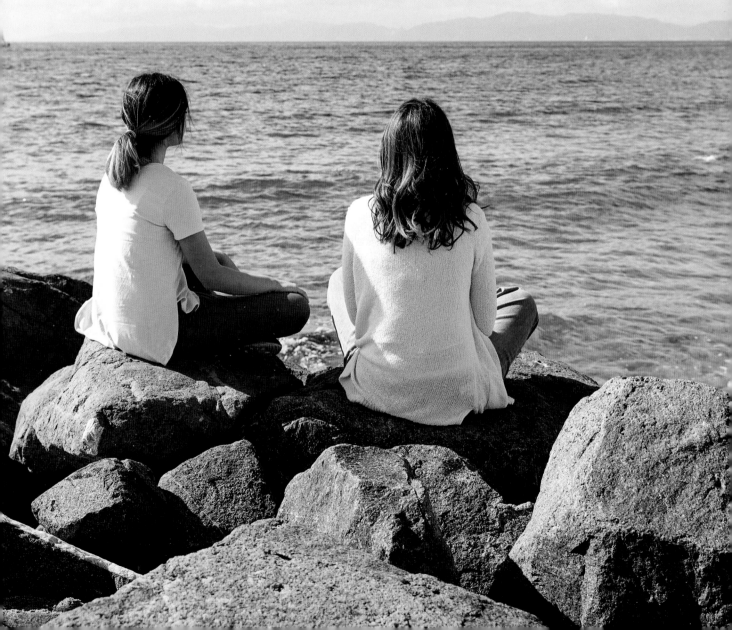

To Alex and Sophie

With this book we hope to leave them a more peaceful, compassionate, and healthier world, filled with taste, beauty, and passion.

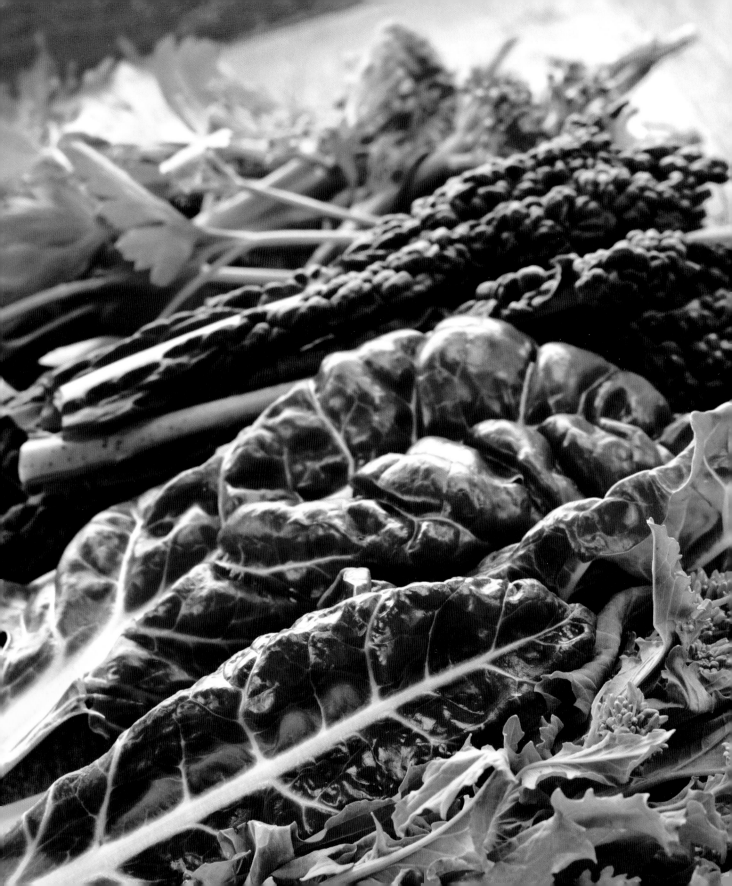

Contents

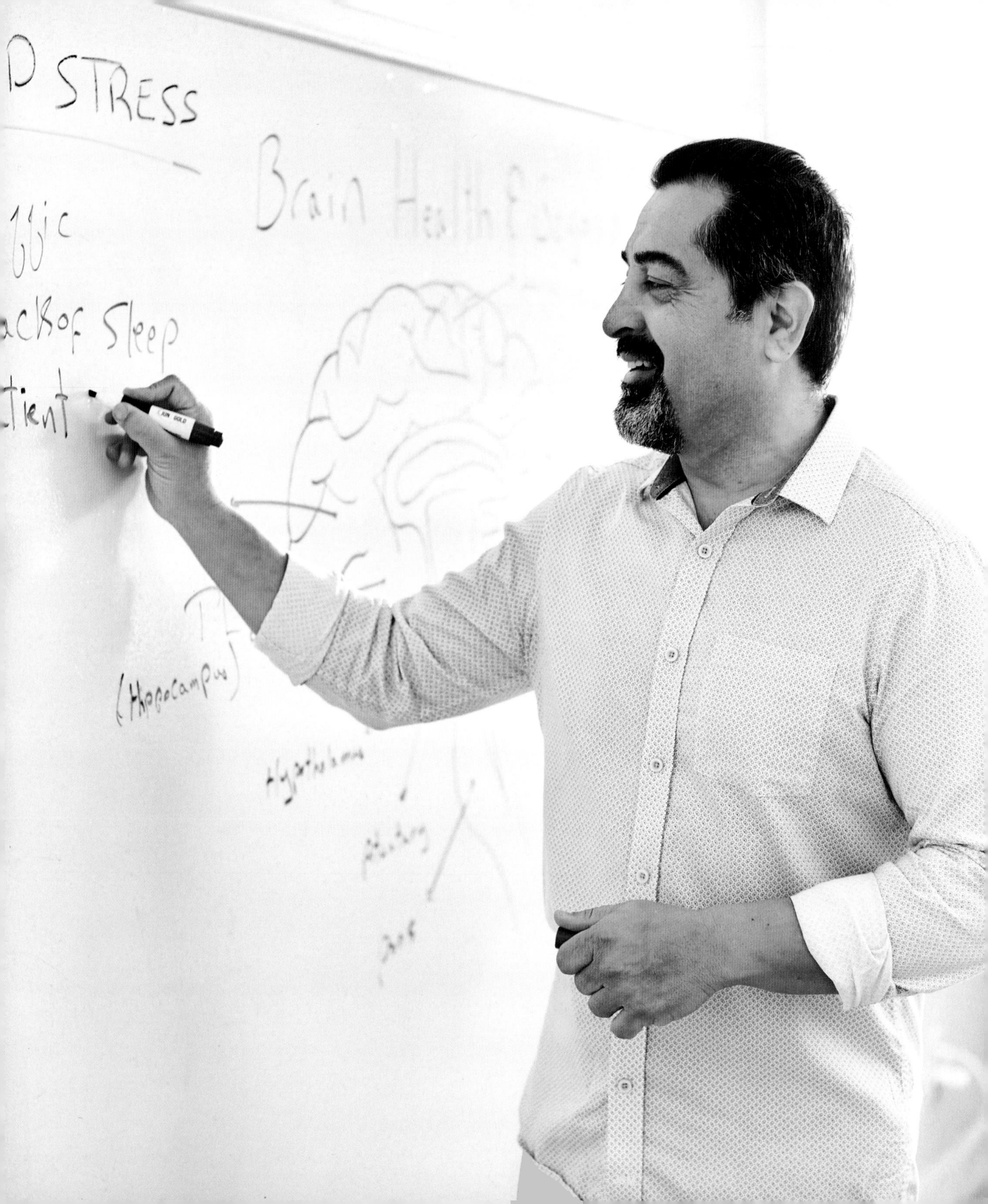
STRESS
Brain Health
Sleep
(Hippocampus)

Part 1

A PROVEN PLAN FOR ALZHEIMER'S PREVENTION

Your brain processes information and manages your emotions, cognitive function, depression, anxiety, attention—everything. Your brain is who you are—your thoughts and your relationship with yourself.

The brain is the most energy-hungry organ in the human body by far. It consumes 25 percent of your energy and at times up to 50 percent of your oxygen, even while you sleep. Nowadays, with all the technological advances and human progress, it is completely exhausted. Our lives have not gotten any simpler; instead, our lives and especially our minds are overwhelmed—by the hundreds of decisions we must make at work and at home every day; the relentless television programs and news cycle to keep up with; our phones that aren't just used for calls but instead call on us to connect with work, friends, and others 24/7; and so much more. Then there's the fast food that complements the fast life, the kind of food that creates addiction and doesn't in the slightest way meet the high-energy needs of a brain in survival mode. This is food that in the long run is nothing more than poison, despite its short-term survival value.

Put all of this together and the brain is like a home under constant assault from inside and outside.

When we talk about modern brain health, we are addressing issues that didn't even exist for much of the time humans have been around.

If we were to put the course of human evolution into a single day, only the last second of that twenty-four-hour period would represent a lifespan past the age of fifty. Mostly we've been focused on surviving—no one worried about *thriving*. The whole point was not to die before we reproduced; after that, death was fair game. It was simply "run away from tiger, have a baby, then die."

Diets like Paleo harken back to theories about the ways our bodies used to function and how we used to live, but the thing is, we're not doing that anymore! We used to have to run from predators, and that meant we needed quick bursts of energy and a store of fat that we could burn off at short notice—and evolution didn't care about the long-term consequences of a quick, hard burn, because nobody was expected to live past age fifty. But now, instead of surviving, we hope to flourish—and that requires long-term support.

When Dean was in high school, he was captain of the soccer team. He was offered some advice: eat a tablespoon of honey before a game so you get a boost of energy. So Dean bought a container of honey and passed it around to his teammates, everybody eating it by the plastic spoonful.

And during the first fifteen minutes, they killed. They ran like rabbits.

But after that—they were dead. It was as if there wasn't even a team anymore, just a bunch of guys lying on the ground. They never lost a game so badly all year.

Short-term gain is often long-term loss. And when short-term gain comes from high protein and bad fats rather than high fiber, you might achieve both weight loss and energy, but the resulting damage to your neurons due to inflammation and oxidation isn't worth it. No matter how tempting it is to drop all your weight in an instant, through some diet du jour or any other quick fix, don't do it. You'll only harm yourself in the long run.

But it's tempting, we know. For millennia, our neurological system has been primarily driven by the part of our brain called the amygdala, which is trained to watch out for "tigers." It has done its job very well; but now, we need to get out of our amygdala, from that emergency state of mind, into the frontal lobe, the control panel of our personality that gives us the ability to communicate and function at a higher level. But the frontal lobe needs our support. We are powering our brains with the kind of food—bad fats, refined sugars, and excessive salt—that's just not sustainable for a healthy brain.

debilitating disease. Concentration, memory, focus, creativity, and productivity—all these are suffering as our brains struggle to keep up with the demands we place on them. There are also related issues, such as the rise in other dementias and stroke, as well as depression and anxiety—something a whopping 17.3 million people in the United States struggle with.[1]

We know this is a lot to process. But there's good news.

The brain is incredibly resilient. Your brain has approximately eighty-seven billion neurons and as many as one quadrillion neural connections, all interacting every moment of every day. Your cells rejuvenate, resist damage, and support growth—at any age. Your neurons can make as few as two connections, or as many as thirty thousand; you have the ability to improve your brain function, to increase your neural connectivity—we'll suggest ways you can do this—to protect yourself against most degenerative, vascular, and inflammatory diseases of the brain.

Better yet, you can profoundly improve your brain function starting right now.

Nearly six million people are living with Alzheimer's disease in the United States alone, and that number is increasing. And that's not even the worst of it. In the general population, brain function is going downhill even without that

Imagine a family sitting around the dinner table. On one night this family gets takeout fried chicken, with each member having a side of medium fries, coleslaw, and a 16-ounce soft drink. There are as many calories in this meal as in the caloric requirement of *each day*, with almost 60 grams of saturated fats, more than 3 grams of sodium, and 65 grams of added sugar—all of which you don't need. Everybody is sitting together at the table, but no one is talking. Instead, they're each on their phones, scrolling away. At the end of the meal, they're tired and collapse in front of the television.

Calling this a "food coma" isn't far from the truth! This dinner has put their brains through shock, and they are going into "postprandial narcolepsy"—an after-dinner sleepiness— because the blood supply and energy regulation of the brain is overwhelmed. This soporific effect of a meal—which we have all felt at one time or another—is common, but that doesn't mean it's good. It's an overwhelm of the system.

Now imagine the same family having dinner the next night. They are eating a home-cooked meal that is high in nutrients. They're paying attention to the various flavors—umami (savory taste), brightness, tanginess—and enjoying the pleasures of a variety of vegetables, some pine nuts, and some berries. Light music plays in the background, and they are engaged in conversation, discussing mutual interests, the challenges of their day, laughing with one another. At the end of the meal, they are energized. They want to go for a walk, look at the stars, play a board game, and continue their dialogue—one that was strengthening their mental functioning without any concerted effort.

The first meal was harmful. The second one was healing.

What happened on the second day is something we call the NEURO BOOST, a positive outcome based on the NEURO PLAN, our five-pronged approach to improving cognitive health, as well as overall health. NEURO stands for

N—Nutrition
E—Exercise
U—Unwind
R—Restore
O—Optimize

And the very first thing to address is Nutrition.

N IS FOR NUTRITION

With every meal you eat, you either make or break your brain. You choose, with every bite, which direction to tilt the needle. Each of the two meals the above family ate had a profound and lasting effect on their overall health, but particularly their brain health. The good news here is that if every meal can damage, then every meal can heal. That's the power of food. We can move beyond simply consuming calories for survival.

This book is about the joy of building cognitive capacity with each meal.

Your brain function is under your control. If you follow our NEURO Plan, here's what you can expect:

SHARPER FOCUS. Focus is the foundation of all consciousness. It determines how quickly you process information or commit something to memory—or whether you can process anything at all. Once you create a system where your brain is no longer overstimulated or inflamed, your ability to focus will escalate exponentially. This happens *almost immediately* after you begin the NEURO Plan.

DISEASE PREVENTION. We're not talking about just Alzheimer's disease. Most chronic neurological diseases—stroke, migraine, diabetic neuropathy—are associated with metabolic processes that are susceptible to environmental factors. You will be at least 80 to 90 percent less likely to have a stroke, with a 90 percent reduced risk for Alzheimer's within a normal lifespan, as extrapolated from the studies on the relationship of lifestyle factors and genetics. Yes, we're talking a *90 percent reduction.*

STRONGER IMMUNE SYSTEM. The part of your brain that regulates your emotions is directly connected to your hypothalamus through your limbic system. If the hypothalamus receives stress from the limbic system, it passes it along to the pituitary, which together with the hypothalamus is responsible for hormone regulation. If the pituitary gets stressed, it releases chemicals that cause your endocrine and immunological systems to go haywire. But once you've got your amygdala and limbic system calmed down, your immune system will be able to operate in an optimal state. You'll have a lot less stress, which means a lower chance of developing infections and disease.

HIGHER MENTAL PROCESSING SPEEDS. Imagine being able to solve problems faster, access your stored memories more quickly, and complete projects at a greater speed than you ever thought possible.

BETTER MEMORY. Inflammation is the body's response to injury. When your brain is inflamed, your ability to form short-term memories is impaired, as is your ability to connect those memories to islands of long-term memory. As inflammation is reduced, both your short-term and long-term memory will improve within the first few weeks of the NEURO Plan.

MORE CREATIVITY. Right now, your amygdala and limbic system are probably overstimulated and therefore overactive, keeping you in fight-or-flight mode. As they calm down, your frontal and parietal lobes can take center stage, allowing you to bring more creativity and control to the way you see the world around you and to the choices you make.

GREATER PRODUCTIVITY. Microglia, the janitor cells of the brain, are nine to ten times more numerous than neurons, and they've got a really important job. While you're sleeping, they prune bad connections between neurons and eliminate the waste products created during the day, but just one night's bad sleep can cause them to eat away at good brain connections. Once you've created a clean system with all neurons firing, however, and an environment within your body that invites restorative sleep, your brain will transform into an efficient, smooth-running machine. Eating the right foods can help you improve your sleep, which will then help the microglia to function better—which will then improve your sleep even more and repair the brain. It's a wonderful circle of health.

BETTER SLEEP. Poor sleep is caused by indigestion, stress from the day, and improper energy metabolism, among many other factors. A diet high in processed sugar and bad fats causes quick, high energy, which prevents you from sleeping well, and a sudden drop in glucose while you're sleeping may cause nightmares. Our suggestion of eating complex carbohydrates before sleep will give your body even energy levels throughout the night so that you aren't plateauing and peaking, being overstimulated or understimulated. And as you sleep better over time, hey, guess what? Your brain works better, too.

HIGHER INTELLIGENCE. Yes, you read that right. If you follow the NEURO Plan, you will be—in a word—sharper. Most people spend very little time actually thinking in a way that engages their frontal lobe and higher cortical centers. We can't maintain focus because our damaged brains can make it literally painful to concentrate. So we coast along, moving from habitual thought to habitual thought, never pinpointing, clarifying, or working through a goal or problem or long-term plan in an unclouded way. But once you unleash the kraken of the higher brain centers like the prefrontal cortex, you'll break those patterns and move into . . . well, a more complex and organized way of thinking. We're talking about something we call XQ: EXTRAORDINARY QUOTIENT. Once you actively build your processing speed, you can focus at a higher and more youthful level. You know how children are capable of learning languages with an ease adults cannot achieve? You'll rediscover and reclaim that. You'll exist at higher cognitive states—that's XQ.

OVERALL HAPPINESS. Inflammation, as well as glucose and fat dysregulation that results from poor food choices, can tap into the baseline survival and anxiety-driven centers of the brain. If this pattern continues for days, weeks, or months, it can result in a baseline anxious and depressed mental state. But if you take away inflammation, and remedy the damage done through highly processed foods, and instead provide the brain with a stable and efficient source of energy from unprocessed, clean, high-nutrient foods, it becomes much easier to reduce anxiety and depression.

Your neurotransmitters, rather than firing in a chaotic, anxiety-producing pattern, will find a stable state, or homeostasis, in a pattern that will promote happiness and a sense of peace.

SUPERHUMAN CALM. The amygdala, the center of all your emotions, is not a complex behavior processor. It is a reactive organ, and it's affected by everything, particularly your hormones and energy levels. It's pretty much a toddler. And when it's inflamed, it's more powerful than the rest of the brain and shouts over everything else. Think of your amygdala as the Hulk. But once you've got that Bruce Banner of a frontal lobe back in charge, your amygdala will pipe down and you'll be able to respond to situations with more reason, less reactivity, and a more even temper.

WEIGHT LOSS. You will lose weight if you need to when you follow the NEURO Plan. Better still, weight loss will happen in a stable way—no more fluctuations after a certain point. If you maintain the NEURO Plan diet and lifestyle, your body will land at its appropriate weight, and stay there.

Promises, Promises

So that's a lot of promises. But we're scientists and researchers, and we don't make promises like that unless we are 100 percent certain they are backed up by research and experience. We have a vibrant community of patients and friends following our NEURO Plan with amazing results.

We began this journey fifteen years ago, when we decided that we needed to become experts in preventing cognitive decline—something that was entirely unheard of at the time! Ayesha did dual residencies in both preventive medicine and neurology before going on to study epidemiology and vascular diseases of the brain at Columbia University, again focusing on prevention.

Dean undertook molecular research and ran clinical trials at the University of California at San Diego as well as at the National Institutes of Health before deciding to move to Loma Linda, California, where he could focus more specifically on clinical work. At Loma Linda, we were able to collect data on three thousand people and study their lifestyles, which allowed us to do significant work on lifestyle epidemiology and how it can impact cognitive decline, especially Alzheimer's. We didn't just look at dementia in our clinic or through various secondary databases of other populations—we went to our local communities and talked to people, which is how we were able to identify factors that contribute to cognitive decline as well as get a sense of the awareness these communities had around cognitive health.

We are uniquely positioned to offer this kind of support, as we are the only physicians who have led molecular research projects, run clinical trials, and organized community-based interventions in this field. At the beginning of our careers, when we first highlighted the impact of lifestyle on brain health, it was not accepted that lifestyle could affect cognition—or that dementia could be prevented. By 2017, when our first book, *The Alzheimer's Solution*, came out, people were finally starting to accept what we had known for years—and now, it's almost universally understood that lifestyle has a significant effect on cognitive decline and dementia.

We're so proud that this concept emerged from our research. Our nonprofit organization, the Healthy Minds Initiative, has been working to raise awareness in communities across the United States, demystifying the steps required to achieve long-term brain health. We are teaching how to prevent devastating illnesses such as Alzheimer's and dementia—and people are making it happen. It's incredible to watch this change in attitude.

.... 99 ....

A couple of years ago I was diagnosed with mild cognitive impairment . . . I can actually feel the difference that these thirty days have made. My head isn't as cloudy, and it seems as though my thoughts come to me just a little bit better than before.

—MARCUS, AGE FORTY-FIVE

As scientists and researchers, our most important questions are always, Why? and How? Let's start with the why.

The NEURO Plan works because it starts with Nutrition—that is, food. Food is the single greatest tool we have for building better brain health. A brain-healthy diet results in better cognition.

This seems obvious, and yet we find ourselves having to argue for this case again and again. The world accepts the fact that nutrition has an impact on cardiovascular disease and diabetes, but for some reason the brain is treated like it's not a "normal" part of the body, as if it's some magical and mysterious organ that cannot possibly be affected by something as prosaic as food.

The brain is incredible. We're neurologists, so obviously we think the brain does some pretty amazing things. But it's just an organ like any other, and that means food is going to affect it. In fact, food has a much *greater* impact on the brain, because this 3-pound organ can consume more than 25 percent of the body's energy. And given that it is, for the most part, in a hermetically sealed system, because of the blood-brain barrier, it has a hard time getting rid of waste and toxins.

When we fail to nourish our bodies properly, we fail to nourish this energy hog of an organ even more.

What is the best way to nourish the brain? *By eating a variety of unprocessed plant-based foods that have all the macronutrients and micro-*

nutrients that your brain needs without any of the harmful elements.

Although we don't believe in reductionism, and we believe you should simply focus on eating a whole-food, plant-based diet, there are some foods that you need to consume every day. We've narrowed them down to nine high-impact brain foods.

The NEURO 9

These nine foods are crucial for maintaining and improving your cognitive health, and you should eat them every single day. The serving size we're suggesting is the *minimum* intake you should be getting while following the NEURO Plan.

THE NEURO 9

1. Green Leafy Vegetables	Especially dark green leafy vegetables like kale, watercress, Swiss chard, collard greens, arugula, spinach	3 cups raw or 1.5 cups cooked
2. Whole Grains	Such as oats, quinoa, brown rice, farro, buckwheat	3 servings (½ cup cooked oatmeal, quinoa, brown rice, or 100% whole-wheat pasta is 1 serving)
3. Seeds	Especially ground flaxseeds and chia seeds	2 tablespoons (2 servings)
4. Beans and Legumes	Chickpeas, black beans, pinto beans, lentils, edamame, giant beans, tempeh, tofu	3 servings of ½ cup cooked beans or tofu/tempeh, ¼ cup hummus, or ½ cup peas
5. Berries	Such as blueberries, blackberries, strawberries	½ cup (1 serving)
6. Nuts	Such as walnuts, almonds, cashews	¼ cup (1 serving)
7. Crucifers	Such as broccoli, cauliflower, bok choy, cabbage, Brussels sprouts	1 cup (2 servings)
8. Tea	Green, white, black, or Oolong tea	At least 1 cup daily
9. Herbs and Spices	Especially turmeric, but also sumac, sage, rosemary, thyme, oregano, cloves, Indian gooseberry, saffron	At least ¼ teaspoon daily

How Do You Know What Is Right? Seven Rules

We get it. There's a lot of contradictory information out there regarding nutrition. Is coconut oil good? Should we stick to a Keto diet? This week you read that a plant-based diet is best, but last week you read that you couldn't possibly get enough protein eating like that. Which is it? Everybody is trying so hard to eat a healthy diet, but the definition of "healthy" keeps changing.

It's human nature to want easy answers. If someone says, "Do this relatively easy thing, and you'll be healthy," who wouldn't jump on that train? Particularly if there's "science" to back it up. There have been attempts of late to confuse the issue of health through what's called false equivalency, that is, when a few badly done studies or "well-engineered" (fake) studies are falsely equated with well-designed, valid studies and with more than eighty years and thousands of research articles indicating the exact opposite.

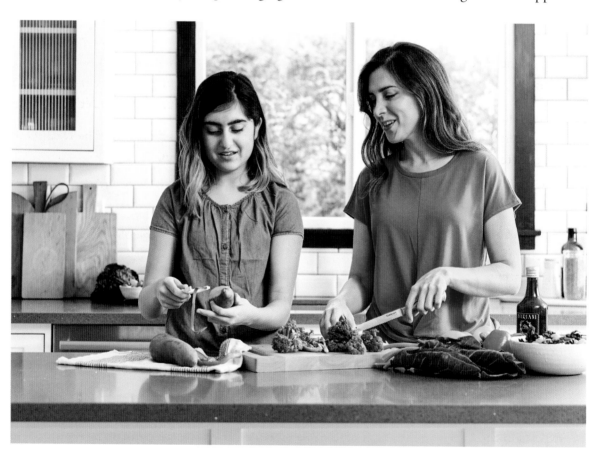

The reality is that nutrition is complex, and there are no easy answers. To be certain that we've got the facts straight, we insist that the research we use and rely on is repeated by others and not biased by funding from those seeking a certain outcome. And we insist on multiple approaches to research, since a different perspective will give different kinds of information. These approaches include:

- **Cross-sectional data,** which look at large populations at one time period

- **Prospective data,** which look at a population followed over a long period of time

- **Retrospective data,** which look back over a long period of time, allowing you to better determine relationships between various factors in an intervention group compared to a control group

- **Randomized clinical trials,** which closely follow the outcomes of a specific intervention

- **Comprehensive review,** including *meta analysis,* which is a systematic way of looking at all the information and research that has been done over a period of time, and coming to a consensus on the work of most of the experts in the field

If all of these approaches, without bias or error, point in the same direction, then we can draw a conclusion. Only then can we have enough confidence to make recommendations to the general public, because understanding nutrition as it applies to diverse populations and across time can be complex. And so, having studied and been involved in all of these different types of research, we are going to take a stand when the conclusion is clear by stating: *This is not an opinion. This is our strongest evidence for public health implementation.*

Based on information that meets our rigorous standards, these are our seven rules for eating your way to a super healthy brain, and they form the foundation of our thirty-day NEURO Plan:

1. **Eat a plant-based diet (and the NEURO 9 foods every day).**

2. **Avoid all foods that are high in saturated fats.**

3. **Avoid refined carbohydrates and sugar.**

4. **Reduce salt and season your food with herbs and spices.**

5. **Avoid processed foods.**

6. **Drink water.**

7. **Eat homemade meals.**

Let's dive into these seven rules a little more closely.

Rule No. 1: Eat a Plant-Based Diet (and the NEURO 9 foods every day)

This is by far the most important of our seven rules. All of the nutrients our bodies need, all of the vitamins and minerals we need for the brain to operate at an optimal level, are found in plants. Plants also contain fiber, which helps create essential short-chain fatty acids in the gut, thus providing potent anti-inflammatory factors for the brain. Plants have everything that's good for you, and if you leave them alone, that is, you don't process them until they are unrecognizable, they are a complete source of nutrients for the brain and the rest of the body.

The same is not true of animal products—meat, poultry, and dairy. Western diets, including what's called the standard American diet (SAD), are typically high in animal products and actively contribute to cognitive decline. One study in Loma Linda, where we see patients and conduct research (Loma Linda is one of the five Blue Zones identified by Dan Buettner where people live the longest and are the healthiest), found that in a group of three thousand individuals, people who ate meat were twice as likely to develop dementia than people who ate a vegetarian diet. Another study in Chicago examined twenty-five hundred participants and found that those who consumed higher amounts of saturated fat from animal products had a higher risk of developing Alzheimer's than those who ate unsaturated fats derived from plants. Adherence to the popular MIND (Mediterranean-DASH Intervention for Neurodegenerative Delay) diet, which is a hybrid of the Mediterranean diet and DASH (Dietary Approaches to Stop Hypertension) diet, has been shown to reduce the risk of Alzheimer's disease by 53 percent. When you look at the components of the MIND diet that are neuroprotective, they are provided by plants, and the diet is low in saturated fats.[2]

WHEN YOU FOLLOW THE NEURO PLAN: You will commit to eating plant-based foods for thirty days straight—eating an abundance of the NEURO 9 and other plant foods (see page 40). You will eat zero meat, dairy, eggs, and fish. This includes shellfish, butter, and cheese.

This is because the meat you are eating is harming your brain. Why is that? Because of the saturated fat content, which leads us right to Rule No. 2.

Rule No. 2: Avoid All Foods That Are High in Saturated Fats

All fats are not equal. There are essential fatty acids and nonessential fatty acids. Essential fats are the ones that your brain needs regularly. They are the "good" fats, polyunsaturated fats (PUFAs), that the body cannot make and are found in plant and marine sources and in some nuts. Nonessential fats are saturated fats and cholesterol that the body can make and does not need, and because they are available in our foods in large amounts, they can cause a lot of damage. The brain contains saturated fats and cholesterol, and it doesn't need it to be restocked!

The requirement is different for newborns and babies, who need some saturated fats when their brains are growing. But for adolescents and adults, the brain simply doesn't need any saturated fats, so all that meat and dairy essentially damage the highways to the brain—the millions of branches of arteries that provide oxygen and nutrition to the energy-hungry brain.

The majority of saturated fats in the typical Western diet come from meats, poultry, and dairy. Saturated fats have been associated with a higher risk of Alzheimer's disease and stroke in multiple high-quality studies, and we are getting the same results over and over again.[3]

There's a lot of confusion about fat consumption in general and brain health, and we'll try to clarify it here without putting you to sleep.

You may hear a lot of self-appointed brain health experts and influencers say that since the brain is about 60 percent fat, you need to eat mostly fat for better brain health. This couldn't be farther from the truth! First of all, the type of fat that makes up the brain is structural fat, which is incorporated in the insulating sheaths of the extensions of neurons, called myelin. These structural fats comprise of different kinds of fats, mostly cholesterol, but this doesn't mean that you have to eat sources of cholesterol, or meat and dairy, to maintain brain health. The brain does not have the capacity to store fat, so you won't find blobs of storage fat like we do in the body. Mind-blowing, isn't it? The brain simply does not have the ability to burn fat as energy like muscles do. Second, the type of fat you're consuming matters. The only types of fat we need are the ones that maintain the integrity of the membranes of the neuron, that is, PUFAs, specifically omega-3 fatty acids.

Saturated fats also cause inflammation, and when they come into contact with our cells, they cause long-term damage, including oxidation. Oxidation happens when a molecule loses an electron, creating what's called a free radical. Free radicals have been shown to cause the microscopic damage ultimately leading to stroke, cancer, heart disease, and other health issues.

For instance, the Women's Health Study conducted at Harvard University determined that women with a diet higher in saturated fat suffered from a faster decline of memory; in fact, they had a 70 percent faster decline in their memory, while women with the lowest saturated fat intake in the study had brains that behaved as if they were six years younger.[4]

The big point of confusion around saturated fats is this: some people think saturated fats are *good* for you. And they're not. The reason for this confusion is because when people stop eating meat and dairy, most of the time they replace it with white bread, white pasta, and other processed foods. Of course that isn't healthy!

If, on the other hand, you replace meat and dairy with beans, vegetables, whole grains, plant-based milks, and nut cheeses, you *will* be healthy—and that's what we're going to help you do. You're going to increase your high-quality plant consumption and replace your saturated fats (which we will refer to as bad fats) with polyunsaturated fats (good fats), which will reduce your risk of developing Alzheimer's and having a stroke and help you build a better brain.

WHEN YOU FOLLOW THE NEURO PLAN: You will avoid all major sources of bad fat, including meat, tropical oils (coconut and palm oils), and dairy, for thirty days. You will get your fats from nuts, seeds, avocados, marine algae, and cold-pressed EVOO and avocado oil (which is predominantly a monounsaturated fat, and in many studies, people who consume extra virgin olive oil instead of other fats such as butter are shown to have a reduced risk of developing brain diseases).

Rule No. 3: Avoid Refined Carbohydrates and Sugar

It's important to remember that the *main and most efficient* source of energy for neurons is glucose, which is the breakdown product of complex carbohydrates found in vegetables, fruits, legumes, and whole grains. Our brains need a constant supply of glucose to function all day long, and this is derived from our food. The brain depends on glucose so much that we have an elaborate receptor system at the blood-brain barrier that allows glucose to quickly pass through and get to the brain.

But the brain needs only a finite amount of glucose to sustain itself. The Western diet is packed with sugar from refined grains and processed foods, and this excess in sugar can damage arteries leading to the brain as well as the various brain structures. Combine that with bad fats and little fiber to regulate glucose release and you've got yourself a toxic concoction ravaging the brain. The brain simply gets too much energy too quickly, forcing the body to work overtime and stressing and overwhelming it at the cellular level.

Remember Dean and the honey and all the team members passing out after the first fifteen minutes? That's what ingesting sugar does to our bodies and brains—and we think nothing of doing it over and over again. Those repeated surges of too much energy cause systemic inflammation, which is linked to cognitive decline. They increase the formation of harmful lipids that thicken and harden artery walls, cutting off the blood supply to the brain. Sugar increases oxidation, which damages cell walls and even DNA. Furthermore, the body needs insulin secreted by the pancreas to help cells take up sugar as a fuel. But when there is too much sugar, the cells become resistant to the insulin, leading to insulin resistance—a condition that severely impairs cells taking up sugar, so it builds up in the blood. This is what causes a lot of damage to the arteries leading to the brain and susceptible structures in the brain like the hippocampus. Our own research has shown that people with insulin resistance have poor cognitive scores on memory tests, even though they aren't diabetic.

And we are consuming more sugar than ever. The American Heart Association recommends no more than 6 teaspoons of added sugar per day for women and 9 teaspoons for men. But we are eating an average of *22* teaspoons per day! The average American consumes a staggering 200 pounds of sugar every year. And unfortunately, most of it is in the refined form—the most dangerous kind. We don't even realize how much sugar we're consuming—or sometimes that we're consuming it at all—because it hides under obscure names like maltose, sucrose, or crystal dextrose and lurks in frightening quantities in foods like pasta sauce, sweetened yogurt, salad dressing, and coleslaw.

WHEN YOU FOLLOW THE NEURO PLAN: You won't eat refined sugar for thirty days. You will eat no white sugar, no honey, no maple syrup, and no agave syrup. You will get more than enough of the glucose your brain needs from eating unrefined plants. For those of you with a sweet tooth, we have some recommended whole-food swaps you can use, along with some amazing recipes that use date paste, blended fruits, and monk fruit sweetener to tame those cravings!

Rule No. 4: Reduce Salt and Season Your Food with Herbs and Spices

Sodium found naturally in foods in the right quantity isn't bad. The two elements in salt, sodium and chloride, are essential to our diets. They help with fluid balance, nerve conduction, and muscle contraction; they're part of normal functioning in every single cell in the body.

The problem is that so much salt is added to our food as an unnecessary flavoring, as well as a preservative. It is shocking how much added salt we get in our diet every day. Too much salt can impair blood pressure, and especially cerebral blood flow, which damages the larger blood vessels leading to the brain (called atherosclerosis) and blowing out the smaller blood vessels that enter the substance of the brain by the millions. This leads to impediments to the blood flow to critical brain structures and micro-bleeds and other forms of vascular damage, which we see in our patients' brain imaging studies every day—individuals in their forties and fifties with dozens of lesions in the deep parts of the brain. These lesions are vaguely called things like "white matter disease" and don't get recorded as strokes in medical records, but they result in memory and attention problems and subsequent cognitive decline. It is literally an epidemic in this population—ubiquitous, but never discussed.

Also, people who consume a lot of salt tend to have damaged arteries in the rest of the body, which manifests as high blood pressure. High blood pressure has been found to be closely associated with vascular dementia and Alzheimer's, as well as other types of brain diseases like stroke.

Herbs and spices not only pack a ton of flavor, they are an easy way of adding potent anti-inflammatory and antioxidant compounds to your diet. Many of the herbs and spices we use, such as cilantro, rosemary, sage, turmeric, thyme, and oregano, have been used for their medicinal properties for thousands of years and are hugely beneficial to the entire body but are particularly necessary for the brain. The standard American diet creates a huge prob-

lem with the efficient clearance and reduction of inflammatory by-products, and herbs and spices can help mitigate this to some extent. They contain high amounts of potent antioxidant compounds that fight oxidative damage in the brain, some even matching the effectiveness of some anti-inflammatory drugs and boosting the immune system.

We recommend consuming herbs and spices regularly. Spices are essentially dried fresh herbs or roots, while herbs can be consumed fresh or dried. Consider turmeric: this seemingly humble spice has been associated with a reduced load of amyloid proteins. It appears that curcumin, a component of turmeric, can bind to amyloid plaque, after which such plaque is recognized by the immune system and removed. Wouldn't it be wonderful if we started thinking of our spice rack as a medicine cabinet?

WHEN YOU FOLLOW THE NEURO PLAN: You will learn to love your spice rack, especially those high-flavor, high-impact spices like cumin, paprika, coriander, sumac, and turmeric; and you will discover a love you never knew for herbs like parsley, basil, thyme, mint, and oregano.

Rule No. 5: Avoid Processed Foods

First, let's start with the definition of processed food. A processed food is the result of starting with a regular food, like wheat, and taking things away from it and adding things to it until it becomes, say, a Wheat Thin. In creating a Wheat Thin, much of the fiber, potassium, B vitamins, protein, iron, riboflavin, and thiamine in wheat are stripped away, and bad fats, preservatives, sugar, and salt replace them.

Processed foods give us more calories for less nutritional value—the opposite of more bang for your buck. And because our food has become so highly processed and refined, we've lost track of how real food looks and tastes. To increase "palatability," salt, sugar, artificial coloring and scent, and several other chemicals have been added to foods for decades. And as we've gotten used to such flavors, manufacturers increase amounts of salt, fat, and sugar until the quantities are literally toxic.

More than that, we are removing nutrients and adding chemicals to give a product a longer shelf life. Many have been around for only a short time, and we have no idea what the long-term effects of consuming them will be. The artificial nature of all of this—too much salt, too much sugar, too much fat, and too few nutrients—has created a kind of negative synergy. The toxic combination is much worse than any one thing on its own.

Real, whole foods that you prepare or cook yourself will fuel your body and brain.

WHEN YOU FOLLOW THE NEURO PLAN: You will eat real food. You won't be shopping for premade food or any kind of packaged food.

Instead, you'll get comfortable in the kitchen and find joy in cooking food that you know is good for you.

Rule No. 6: Drink Water

Water should be your main beverage. It can be tap, mineral, or carbonated water. We recommend drinking eight to ten glasses of clean, refreshing water every day.

Don't drink juice. Juice is in fact a processed food: you've taken a whole-plant food and removed its fiber and nutrients until you're left with nothing but water and sugar and maybe a few vitamins. Don't drink soda, energy drinks, sugary flavored water—any of that stuff. Just drink water.

We recommend that you *not* drink alcohol during the thirty days of the NEURO Plan. Alcohol is a sugar-based product, so it's already not great—but it gets worse. The data on alcohol and brain health point to the health benefits of reducing alcohol as much as possible. Excessive drinking has been linked to an increased risk of dementia, and even moderate drinking—defined as no more than one drink a day for women and two for men—is associated with shrinking in the areas of the brain associated with cognition and learning. In a recent British study, participants who consumed the equivalent of four or more drinks a day had almost six times the risk of hippocampal shrinkage as nondrinkers, while moderate drinkers had three times the risk.[5]

You've probably heard about the benefits of a compound called resveratrol, which is found in red wine, and its lifespan-increasing properties. But the amount of red wine you'd have to drink to get a sufficient quantity—thousands of glasses—would damage your body severely. No thanks. Get your resveratrol from grapes, blueberries, and cocoa.

When you're young, your body is 70 to 75 percent water, but as you age, you lose water from all tissues. Changes in cellular structure mean that cells can no longer hold on to water molecules, and the connective tissues between those cells also atrophy. This isn't helped by the fact that as we age we retain fewer fluids. We also tend to have a decreased sense of thirst (though we need just as much water as ever), which exacerbates the issue.

Water serves multiple functions: it regulates temperature, it provides flow for electrolytes and the lymphatic and blood systems, and, crucially for brain health, it provides a cushion. A jogging person who is dehydrated can slam his or her brain against the surrounding bony structures without that cushion. Even small movements can cause microtraumas in the brain if you aren't properly hydrated. And a loss of as little as 2 to 3 percent of water in the elderly can cause cognitive impairment. Those eight to ten glasses of water a day are crucial.

And as we said, it doesn't have to be plain water. Carbonated water is fine, as long as it doesn't have added chemicals or sugars.

Be wary of drinking tea instead of water. Tea is wonderful for brain health, especially green tea (one of our NEURO 9), but it can act as a diuretic, especially if it's high in caffeine, leading to dehydration.

The same applies for coffee, as it has a diuretic effect, too. Coffee is a concentrated source of antioxidants, and some literature shows modest benefits among coffee drinkers such as lower rates of dementia—but only if they don't have heart disease and/or psychological problems like sleep disorders or anxiety, and only if they are consuming filtered coffee (filters remove a compound called cafestol, which can increase blood lipid levels). Also, stay away from cream and sugar and substitute plant milk and monk fruit sweetener instead.

WHEN YOU FOLLOW THE NEURO PLAN: You will drink a lot of water. You'll come to crave it even more than your accustomed daily drink, whether that's a glass of wine or a diet cola.

Rule No. 7: Eat Homemade Meals

You are going to learn how to gain control over what you eat. The truth is that health is not found in a clinic or a hospital—it is attained and sustained at home, at work, and in the community. If you cook your own food at home, you will become physically familiar with your food, you will learn what works for your body and what doesn't, and you will be able to overcome all the limitations that usually stop people from becoming healthy and staying that way.

When we eat out, we don't really know what we're eating. At best, we get a one-sentence description on the menu that doesn't tell us much of anything at all. Restaurants use staggering amounts of salt, sugar, and bad fats in their foods, and we simply can't know how much we're getting. Order a salad at a restaurant and you feel like you're doing a great job—but it turns out that salad may contain 4 grams of saturated fat, 9 grams of added sugar, and a whopping 1,010 milligrams of sodium. (Compare that with our Kale Fennel Seed Salad [page 201], which has 0.8 grams of saturated fat, no added sugar, and 176 milligrams of sodium.)

When you cook at home, you can skip the bad fat and refined added sugar and use only the salt you truly need—which you will quickly discover isn't anywhere near as much as you are used to! Your palate will change as you get used to being able to taste your *food*, not the sugar, salt, and fat used to "flavor" it. You will eat cleaner, more nutritious food.

We recently put in an herb garden, and it was a revelatory moment. When Dean picked thyme for the first time and crushed it between his fingers, the scent burst out, and it was spectacular. So much flavor is available, and when you cook with those flavors yourself, it becomes real, and it becomes *yours.* You have the power to make delicious food. It's not some secret that only chefs can know—*anyone* can do it, because the flavors and ingredients are available to all of us! And not only do herbs taste good, they are good *for* you. These tiny, fragrant, savory plants are not only flavoring your food, they're actually healing you. An herb garden is a medicine garden, and it's a form of medicine that is natural and real.

Try to grow your own small herb and vegetable garden. You'll be surprised at how easy it can be and, with some creative gardening, how little space you need. We've got some ideas for you on our website (teamsherzai.com), and we think you'll be pleasantly surprised by how calming a small garden can be. And whether you grow your own food or not, cooking it for yourself is exciting, creative, and empowering.

WHEN YOU FOLLOW THE NEURO PLAN: You will become a home chef! You will eat fresh, natural, and brain-healthy foods, and you'll probably find that they taste better.

WHAT ABOUT THE REST OF NEURO?

We've talked about the N in NEURO—Nutrition. It's the most important part, the most efficient first step. But it's not the only part. Your

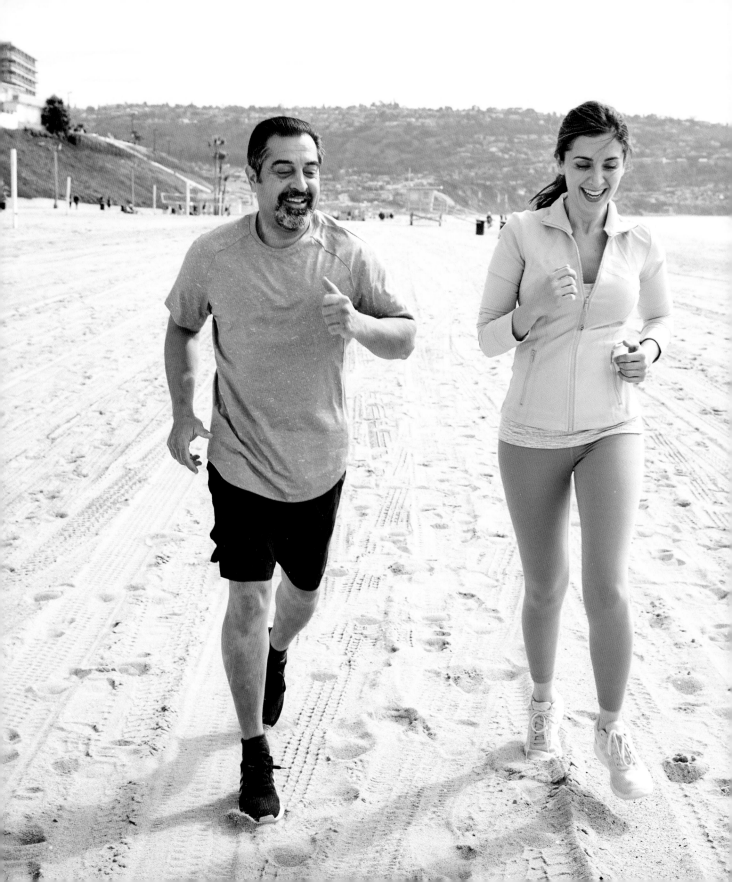

diet alone won't do it, because contrary to what you've heard, you aren't just what you eat. You're also what you do, and how you recover from all that doing. It's all bound together, with nutrition supporting everything in a wonderfully synergistic way. To achieve true brain health, you have to support your diet with the rest of NEURO: Exercise, Unwind, Restore, and Optimize.

E Is for Exercise

We know you've heard this before. Breaking news: exercise is good for you! But the thing is, it really, *really* is. And not just for cardiovascular health, although that's true, or mental health, although that's also true, but very specifically for brain health. Regular exercise reduces inflammation and oxidative processes, so that if you eat an unhealthy meal, exercise will help you create an environment that reduces the damage caused by that meal. Now this doesn't mean you should go out and eat a bunch of processed food and think that if you run a mile afterward you've done your brain any favors. You haven't. You've just made the processed food a little less damaging.

Exercise—which we define as both aerobic exercise and strength training—has an enormous impact on brain health, automatically boosting cognitive function by increasing blood flow and combating clogged arteries, vascular stiffness, insulin resistance, and high cholesterol. Long periods of inactivity mean less blood makes its way to your brain.

Imagine a conversation with a co-worker about a project you're working on. The deadline is approaching, and you ask your co-worker how to do a specific task. That person explains it to you, and you even watch over his or her shoulder to see how it's done. You feel like you've got it, and so you say thank you and head back to your desk. But on your way, you stop and get some water, take a quick personal call, and by the time you're sitting back at your computer, you've completely forgotten everything your co-worker told you. *How do I do that task, again?*

We've all had this experience. As our brains age, we lose neurons and the connections between them, and short-term memories like these become harder to hold on to. Exercise can slow that loss and enhance that connectivity, no matter how old you are. Those connections are particularly important for the medial temporal lobe, the part of your brain responsible for short-term memory and its conversion to long-term memory. Aerobic and strength activities boost both the number and viability of those connections, providing stronger, more plentiful hooks to hang that memory on. Exercise also helps the various parts of the brain communicate with each other because it improves the integrity of the white matter tracts of the brain. Best of all, with regular exercise, you can grow millions of new brain connections, even late in life.

The good news is that you don't need to run a marathon to have a healthy brain. Something as simple as a daily brisk walk and a few squats can lower your risk of Alzheimer's by 40 percent. Exercise doesn't have to be a burden. It can be simple and definitely enjoyable, and we will show you how to make it work for you.

WHEN YOU FOLLOW THE NEURO PLAN: You will do moderate but targeted exercise, focusing on strength-building, cardio, and flexibility. You'll exercise in a way that's right for *your* body.

U Is for Unwind

It's important to understand that there are two kinds of stress. Normally when we talk about stress, we're talking about the bad kind—the kind that keeps you from sleeping and can raise blood pressure. But there is also good stress— the kind you experience when working toward a life goal or succeeding at a project at work or at home. Stress affects your hormone levels, and with positive stress, your oxytocin levels go up, your cortisol and adrenaline levels go down, and your frontal lobe is engaged. This kind of stress actually improves your brain function.

But, as we've all experienced, bad stress— uncontrolled stress—sends your brain function into a spiral of hormonal, neurotransmitter, and immunological chaos. It alters your dopamine

and serotonin levels, causing increased anxiety and depression. It does the opposite of what good stress can do for you: it increases your cortisol and adrenaline levels, causes aberrations in your thyroid and growth hormones, and even causes changes in your insulin levels and immune system. It directly affects the billions of connections between the neurons, which in turn affects your concentration, attention, decision-making, judgment, and memory formation. And it literally causes your brain to shrink, as it inhibits the production of neuronal and axonal growth hormones. At the same time, the negative effect of bad stress on your brain's glial cells causes them to start attacking perfectly good brain structures and cells, especially in vulnerable areas like the hippocampus, the part of your brain responsible for memory. Uncontrolled long-term bad stress also negatively impacts your immune system, weight, heart rate, and blood pressure.

All of this happens because bad stress puts the body into autonomic overdrive, which increases cortisol, a stress hormone produced by the adrenal gland. Cortisol is intended for that run-away-from-a-tiger moment, spiking your blood glucose levels and giving you a burst of energy. But those higher levels cause considerable long-term damage; all of the above issues come down to a long-term excess of cortisol.

When you are under this kind of stress, it affects your hunger centers, and your satiety can go way up, or way down, so that you're either overeating or barely eating at all. Either way, your relationship with food is negatively impacted, and your body's pituitary/endocrine system doesn't allow you to metabolize the food you do consume—and that food is most often sugary or fatty, because this kind of stress makes your amygdala choose the short-term foods that could help you survive that stress.

Getting the amygdala to calm down is a two-step process. The simplest step (though by no means the easiest) is to deny it those sugary, fatty foods it craves. But you have to support that by working to bring your stress levels down. Start by identifying your bad stressors and actively work to reduce or eliminate them as much as you can. Then identify the good stressors and systematically work to make them a central part of your life. Meditation, exercise, yoga, listening to music, decluttering your environment, cultivating healthy relationships, and especially living a purpose-driven life have all been scientifically shown to dramatically reduce uncontrolled stress.

But remember, you don't want to reduce all stress. The good stress that comes from pursuing long-term goals toward an important milestone (like, for example, finding that purpose-driven life) helps make your brain more resilient and allows your higher cortical function, particularly the frontal lobe, to take center stage. When this happens, your thinking brain can control the emotional brain, curbing its cravings for sur-vival foods and instead inspiring you to seek the kinds of foods that help you survive in the long term—nutrient-rich, sustaining, healing foods. Those healing foods in turn will enhance the parts of the brain that maintain higher cognitive function and focus with good stress and reduce the activity of the fight-or-flight system driven by bad stress.

WHEN YOU FOLLOW THE NEURO PLAN: You will identify your stressors and practice methods of relieving bad stress such as meditation, mindful breathing, listening to music, journaling, and engaging in a variety of practices that will help you find a sense of calm.

R Is for Restore

Restorative sleep is absolutely critical to good health. The entire body benefits from restorative sleep, but this highly risky activity (which basically puts the body in a vulnerable, paralyzed state for many hours of the day) is something we do mostly for the sake of our brains. For the brain, sleep is a super spa. While you are sleeping, your brain enters a completely different metabolic and processing state; in fact, your brain does some of its most impressive work during this time.

We now know that during sleep, the brain takes care of two immensely important house-keeping tasks. First, it is removing the day's cumulative waste, including inflammatory and oxidative products and all the other abnormal proteins and toxins that accumulate. Second, the brain is converting short-term memories into long-term memories, getting rid of useless ones like a jingle you heard on the radio; organizing thought processes; and building new connections throughout the brain. With restorative sleep, you are happier, more focused, more coordinated, and basically smarter (by as much as 40 to 60 percent), as well as less likely to have headaches and strokes and more likely to have regulated weight and a significantly improved libido.

Here's how this happens. Restorative sleep is characterized by non-rapid eye movement (NREM) and rapid eye movement (REM) sleep. NREM sleep is divided into three stages: stage one is light sleep, during which you can be easily awakened; stage two is deeper, when your memory begins to be consolidated; and stage three is what we call slow-wave sleep, during which memory consolidation peaks. Sufficient amounts of slow-wave sleep allow for greater memory retention.

During REM sleep, the brain organizes information and restructures itself, kind of like defragging a hard drive. This allows for greater concentration, focus, creativity, reason—all the benefits of a high-functioning brain.

The problem is that many of us have trouble achieving sleep beyond stages one or two and don't cycle through these stages properly. When this happens, we experience "brain fog." Our limbic system is affected. The frontal lobe is weakened. We feel tired. Our emotions are out of control, and we crave food even when we're not hungry— because the body is trying to provide us with the energy we didn't get from sleep. Sleep deprivation leads to significant changes in key opposing hormones in appetite regulation: leptin and ghrelin. These hormones bind to the hypothalamus of the brain and suppress (leptin) or stimulate (ghrelin) the appetite. Sleep deprivation reduces the effects of leptin and increases our sensitivity to ghrelin, leading to hunger irrespective of food consumed and weight gain. The amygdala has gone into survival mode again, urging us to select foods that are calorie-rich and often nutrient-poor—which of course makes everything worse, as all that sugar or fat makes it harder for us to sleep, and the vicious cycle continues.

It is possible to break this pattern, but it will take some patience and effort on your part. Certain foods will help you sleep better, but *when* you eat matters as much as what you eat. Active digesting prevents restorative sleep, so make sure you allow your body plenty of time to work through a meal before going to bed—or better yet, don't eat high-energy foods within two to three hours before sleep.

It's also a question of circadian rhythms, the body's innate twenty-four-hour biological processes. When we're exposed to daylight, the pineal gland starts producing melatonin, the sleep hormone. When the sun goes down, it releases that melatonin, usually around 9:00 p.m. By 9:00 a.m., those levels fall and we become alert. It's a pretty simple system. But any disruption in light exposure throws the whole system off. Chronic disruption of circadian rhythms has been shown to have a cumulative negative effect on cognitive function, and completely alters our relationship with food.

We will help you eat, exercise, and time your life to set yourself up to achieve good, restorative sleep.

WHEN YOU FOLLOW THE NEURO PLAN: You will learn some "best practices" for getting a good night's sleep, including going to bed at the right time, waking up at the right time, and avoiding sleep-distorting habits, like looking at TV, phone, tablet, or computer screens before bed.

O Is for Optimize

The kind of good stress we mentioned above, associated with a purpose-driven life, profoundly increases your cognitive reserve. Cognitive reserve is a measure of the connectivity we develop in our brains throughout our lives. A high cognitive reserve means that you are capable of achieving what we have coined your XQ, or EXTRAORDINARY QUOTIENT. Cognitive reserve depends on how much we challenge our brains, how much

information we take in—all the risk, adventure, joy, learning, and experience we accumulate over a lifetime. It is the integrity of the brain, and it is a direct result of how we live our lives. A life well-lived equals a higher cognitive reserve.

Everyone's brain deteriorates as they age, just as everyone's muscles and skin deteriorate. And yet not everyone gets Alzheimer's. Cognitive reserve is about building redundant connections between billions of neurons, as well as redundant connections between brain structures, so that even as the brain ages, it can still function at an optimal level—in fact, at a superoptimal level!

Cognitive reserve is under your control. You can optimize your brain—and therefore protect it—by challenging it. And we mean really challenging it. This isn't going to be as easy as playing a bunch of games of sudoku or doing the Sunday crossword puzzle. Cognitive reserve is built by engaging multiple areas of the brain at once, specifically around your passions, or the things that give you a sense of purpose. Reading a book engages the language centers, which is great. But thinking deeply about what you've read and then discussing it with others engages the frontal lobe, as well as the areas of your brain that respond to language and social interaction.

Multidomain, multifunctional activities like knitting a complex pattern are ideal. Consider how you have to read the instructions, process them, stay focused, understand the spatial properties of the increases and decreases, memorize a pattern repeat, and physically move your hands in the correct way, with the correct tension. You're doing a lot at once—and if you're doing it in the company of others, say in a knitting group, you're also engaging in thoughtful, enjoyable conversation.

That second part, social interaction, is really important. Social engagement is associated with a reduced risk of dementia. People who identify as "lonely" have twice the risk of developing Alzheimer's. In itself, social interaction is a multidomain, multifunctional activity. It engages the brain through facial recognition, memory, focus, attention, auditory skills, and language skills as well as emotional engagement. And when you combine a multidomain cognitive activity with the multidomain activity that is being social, you are giving your brain the most complex activity available. Playing solitaire is one thing. But playing a game of rummy or Hearts with laughter and competition with friends is quite another.

When our food revolves around our social activity, we are healthier. Consider the tradition of "breaking bread" and how that intentional, social interaction around food created trust and bonds between people. The same is true today. If you look at the people who live in the Blue Zones in Loma Linda, Okinawa, Sardinia, Nicoya, and Ikaria, their food consumption is intertwined with their social behavior, and there is a strong sense of community. Loneliness makes people unhealthy, and social interaction and good food together make the ultimate brain support. Incorporating healthy food becomes especially easy if the gathering is intended to promote a Healthy Minds Initiative in your community (if you'll forgive the shameless plug!).

WHEN YOU FOLLOW THE NEURO PLAN: You will spend quality time with friends and family, learn new things, and dive into brain-stretching activities.

THE SUM IS GREATER THAN THE PARTS

If you eat nutrient-rich food, exercise will increase the positive effects of that food. The addition of exercise to good and nutrient-rich food is not additive; it is actually exponential. It's about synergy. We often think of our bodies and our lives as these linear, siloed processes. But they're not; all kinds of things—food, exercise, sleep, stress—add to each other and interact with one another. This is true from a negative perspective as well: as we age, if we're not taking care of ourselves, our bodies break down, and there is a domino effect. For example, when you don't eat a high-nutrient diet, your gut suffers, your bad cholesterol levels go up, and that affects your blood vessels. Once you get plaque deposition, your arteries harden and your heart pumps harder, which can cause abnormal rhythms in the heart and clot formation, leading to a stroke. And a stroke can cause a slew of brain issues. When one thing goes awry, the whole system goes down. But if you eat a high-nutrient diet, you'll get enough fiber and vitamins; your gut will function well, producing better chemicals and metabolizing lipids effectively; and your cholesterol will be low, your blood flow steady, and your brain vibrant.

What is true for your body's pathways is true for every aspect of life. Each of these pillars of health—Nutrition, Exercise, Unwind, Restore, and Optimize—work together to bring you out of the state of survival your body has been in and into a state of growth and vitality. Each part of the NEURO Plan works with the others to create powerful, lasting change. If you follow even just one aspect of the NEURO Plan, your risk of Alzheimer's drops significantly. But if you work with them all together, we believe your risk of developing dementia, stroke, and many other diseases of the brain drops by as much as 80 to 90 percent.

Let's get started!

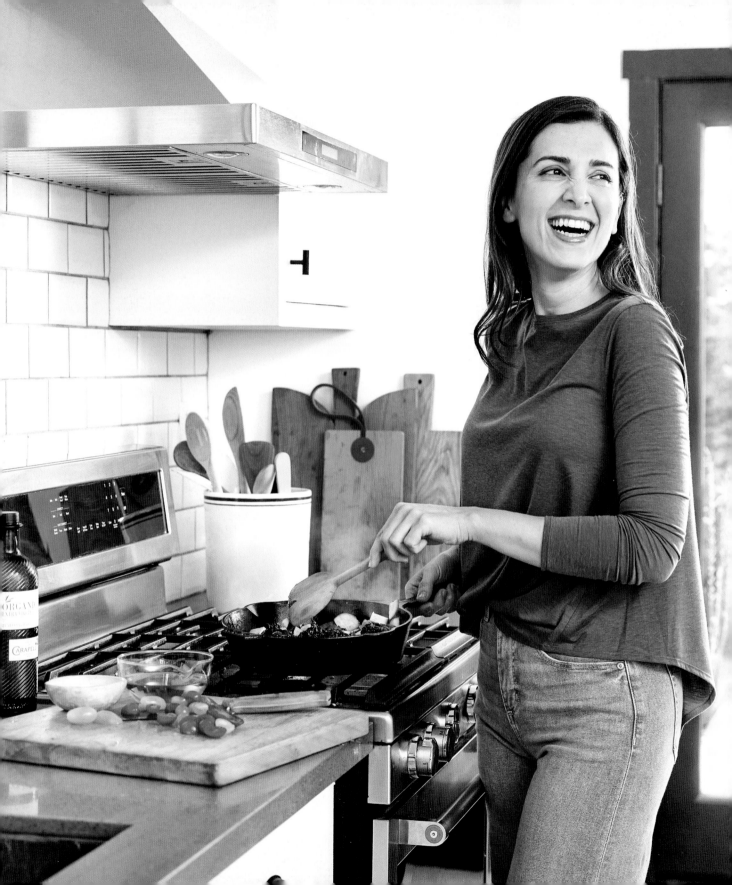

Part 2

WHAT TO EAT, WHAT NOT TO EAT, AND WHY

We know you probably have a lot of questions. We laid down the law pretty strongly there, and we can hear all the protests from here. Honestly, we've howled about them ourselves. "*No meat?!*" cried Dean, back in the day. "*No SUGAR?!*" wailed Ayesha. Even while we were first researching the ways in which nutrition affects the brain, we were still coming up with arguments *against* what we were learning.

It's human nature to protest when something you really, really want is being threatened. But we promise you, we have data-driven reasons for everything we suggest.

NO MEAT. REALLY.

We are serious about this. Don't eat meat. We're not talking about just cutting off the fat or avoiding red meat or eating only fish. *No meat.* At least give it a try for thirty days, and we promise you will see amazing changes.

The reason is quite clear. Meat has saturated fats in its cellular structure that are impossible to eliminate. Simply cutting off the white stuff from your steak won't do it—all that fat is in the red part, too. Even if you ever find "lean meat" without a speck of visible fat in it, it's not going to promote your health. Meat is also high in choline and carnitine, leading to the formation of trimethylamine N-oxide (TMAO) and insulin-like growth factor 1 (IGF-1), which have been associated with heart disease, stroke, cancer, type 2 diabetes, peripheral artery disease, chronic kidney disease, and Alzheimer's—and there are so many more to list.

And what about the "good" white meat? We've been raised to believe that chicken and "the other white meat," pork, are so much better for us than red meat. But it turns out that poultry is actually one of our main sources of saturated fat, because we eat so much of it! One study showed that when participants switched from red meat to white meat, there was *no* significant decrease in their low-density lipoprotein (LDL, or "bad" cholesterol) levels.[6] They also raise the level of TMAO in the body, just like red meat does.

BUT WHAT ABOUT PROTEIN? We've heard it from our patients time and again: "The only way you get protein is by eating meat." This couldn't be farther from the truth. What's the most powerful animal, pound for pound? The gorilla. What does a gorilla eat? Greens. Yes, we do need protein, but it doesn't need to come from meat. In fact, plants are the source of all amino acids, the building blocks of protein, and you don't have to eat another animal to get your protein. Pound for pound, many plant-based foods have as much protein and healthier protein than meat. All of the twenty amino acids can be found in plants. It is absolutely possible to get enough protein from a plant-based diet. And, just as there are good fats and bad fats, there are good proteins and bad proteins. Animal proteins raise your levels of TMAO, which can damage you at the cellular and genetic levels, turning on markers for aging and cancer.

BUT CAN'T YOU GET EVERYTHING YOU NEED FROM A PALEO DIET? Sure, this is true. You can get all your nutrients if you eat meat with your vegetables. But you have to consider what you're getting *with* those nutrients. You wouldn't use a soft drink as your source of water, because while you do get water drinking that soft drink, you also get all kinds of poisons along with it. The same is true for meat. A plant-based diet is a more efficient approach to eating, allowing you to consume your necessary calories in such a way that you get only the positive nutrients, without all the negatives tossed in, too. What's the point of getting iron and protein if you destroy all your arteries along the way? Low-calorie, nutrient-dense foods systematically build the brain rather than destroy it. Plant-based proteins are better for you, because they are free of saturated fats which can damage brain cells and arteries, *plus* you get fiber, vitamins, and minerals along with your protein.

This synergy of nutrients acting together is how you have a well-rounded diet. In fact, a more diverse plate will give you all the nutrients and all the amino acids you need. A plate of French fries by themselves won't provide you with all the nutrients you need, but a dish of beans, greens, and rice will. It's about creating a meal, not looking at just one ingredient.

NOT EVEN FISH?

Plant-based proteins are better than meat, period—and that includes fish. Certainly, studies show that when the standard American diet is adjusted to include more fish, overall brain health improves. Fish is better for you than steak or chicken. But in the most optimal diet for brain health—which translates to all health—you can do even better than that. No evidence suggests that adding fish to a high-quality plant-based diet offers any health benefits at all. And although you don't have to worry about saturated fats when you eat fish, you do have to worry about mercury or lead levels, not to mention other toxic pollutants in water we don't even test for.

All animal meats, including fish, are bio-magnifiers, which means that they accumulate industrial chemicals and toxins as they move higher in the food chain. When a larger predatory fish like tuna ingests a smaller fish that contains mercury, the tuna's mercury levels get even higher as it adds to the mercury it has accumulated from other previously ingested fish. And when people eat an excessive amount of fish (defined as three to four servings per week), particularly large fish like tuna or snapper, their elevated level of methylmercury, which is a highly toxic substance/neurotoxin, causes a lot of damage to the brain and is associated with poor cognitive function. Animals act as a filter for the food they eat, and all fish have some level of mercury. When we eat fish, especially big fish, we are eating the pollutants that they have accumulated in their flesh. Doesn't it strike you as odd that pregnant and breast feeding women are discouraged from eating fish high in mercury because of their child's brain health and growth, and yet it's supposed to be fine for the rest of us? Although this point is disputed, we would rather err on the side of caution.

BUT WHAT ABOUT OMEGA-3 FATTY ACIDS? As we mentioned in Part 1, omega-3 fatty acids are critical for brain health, as they are the foundation of cell membrane function, as well as many other functions in the body. They are the only type of fat that the brain needs to receive daily from outside sources, because our bodies can't make them—they must be derived from food.

There are two classes of essential fatty acids: omega-3s and omega-6s. We need both of them in the right amount for optimal brain function. Omega-6s are found abundantly in our Western diet, but omega-3s are not. The two have essentially opposite effects: omega-6s increase inflammation and the tendency of the blood to clot, and omega-3s lower inflammation and the tendency of the blood to clot. Most people are deficient in omega-3s. The problem is we get way more omega-6s in our typical Western diet than omega-3s, which puts our body into a proinflammatory state. Our goal must be to increase omega-3 and lower omega-6 consumption.

The brain doesn't have any storage fat; it has only structural fat, and that's something the body can make—but remember, it can't make omega-3 fatty acids. As we age, we actually need more omega-3s, and studies have shown that participants with higher levels of omega-3s experienced improved cognitive function, lower rates of brain shrinkage, and overall better brain structure.[7]

Those of you who have explored omega-3s in depth know that there are three main types: short-chain alpha-linolenic acid (ALA) and long-chain eicosapentaenoic acid (EPA) and docosahexaenoic acid (DHA). ALA is found in abundance in nuts and seeds, and the body can convert it to EPA and DHA. Granted, it's at a low rate—only 5 to 15 percent of your ALA will convert to DHA. Some of our favorite NEURO 9 foods are chia seeds and flaxseeds, which have a ratio of omega-3 to omega-6 fatty acids of 3–4 to 1, making them very rare and powerful in the food world.

DHA is the omega-3 that's really important for the brain, and it *is* more easily accessed through eating fish. But the DHA in fish is derived from the algae that fish consume. In order to get direct DHA/EPA, you don't have to eat fish—and it isn't worth it, because who wants all that junk that comes with it? We can get our DHA/EPA from plant-based sources such as flax, chia, and hemp seeds, and other sources. Thanks to better understanding and technology, we can skip the go-between—the fish—and get our DHA/EPA directly from algae omega-3 supplements, without risking the potential neurotoxins.

SIRTUINS

Sirtuins are enzymes that regulate many cellular processes and are related to aging and longevity. Sirtuins (silent information regulators) silence or inhibit certain genes, and when they are suppressed, the process of Alzheimer's disease seems to move much more quickly. Study of the brains of patients with Alzheimer's have revealed that the accumulation of plaques and tangles (the physical evidence of Alzheimer's) is associated with a loss of sirtuin activity.

So what is causing this loss? Advanced glycation end products (AGEs) are toxins that can accelerate aging—and lower sirtuin activity. AGEs are found in high-fat and high-protein

---

Plant-Based Diet Is Not Automatically a Healthy Diet

The first rule of our seven rules for eating your way to a healthy brain (see Part 1) is "eat a plant-based diet." But remember, you can still harm your body and brain if you don't follow the other six rules: avoid saturated and trans fats, avoid refined carbohydrates, reduce salt intake, avoid processed foods, drink water, and eat homemade food. You're not doing yourself any good by skipping the hamburger and going out to eat a whole plate of deep-fried onion rings and French fries instead.

---

foods like chicken, pork, and beef—just another reason to embrace a plant-based diet.

WHAT ABOUT DAIRY?

The issues of saturated fat that we encounter when we eat meat are the same issues we have when we eat dairy. As a matter of fact, dairy is the number one source of saturated fats in the Western diet. And the more concentrated the dairy food, the higher the saturated fats. Cheese is especially high as it is a concentrated form of milk solids.

Be Careful with Kombucha

Touted for its probiotic and antioxidant properties, kombucha is all the rage. But it is often quite high in sugar and contains some alcohol. Most store-purchased brands have a very low alcohol content, but home-brewed kombuchas tend to be higher—*and* there is a higher risk for getting sick, as brewing kombucha is not as straightforward as making a batch of lemonade; it can easily become contaminated with fungi, molds, and unhealthy bacteria.

WHAT ABOUT PROBIOTICS? Probiotics are "good" bacteria; they promote digestive health and boost the immune system. We definitely all need this good gut bacteria, but the question is, do we need to get it from outside sources?

There are a lot of probiotic foods on the market, including kombucha, kefir, sauerkraut, miso, and tempeh, and there are probiotic supplements as well. Some of these have been studied, some haven't. With the over-the-counter supplements, of course, the Food and Drug Administration (FDA) doesn't monitor their manufacture, and so it's not clear whether or not they are high-quality or even if they contain the good bacteria they claim to. It's best to eat foods that can grow the good gut bacteria, which comes from fiber. When gut bacteria break down fiber, they create short-chain fatty acids, which are incredibly protective of gut lining and provide the necessary chemicals, such as butyrate, to act as neuroprotective agents. They also provide alternative fuel for brain cells. Butyrate, for instance, targets many of the pathways that are associated with Alzheimer's and other neurodegenerative diseases like Parkinson's and stroke. Butyrate reduces neuronal death and helps maintain the integrity of the blood-brain barrier.

Fiber is a carbohydrate—that's right, it's a carb!—that has immense health benefits. It nourishes your microbiome *and* your brain. On average, we need at least 30 grams of fiber a day, but only 5 percent of the US population manages to achieve that. We're going to help you get there.

Most of the time, we simply don't know which probiotics are helpful and which are not, or how much is necessary. But the good news is that in a normal, healthy, well-balanced plant-based diet, you don't need to consume probiotics. Instead, you are consuming plenty of *prebiotics*—foods that create an environment that is friendly to probiotics. You don't have to give your body yeast or lactobacillus or bifidobacterium; your body already contains all the friendly microbes it needs, and if you feed them kale and apples and other prebiotics, your microbiome will flourish. Onions, garlic, leeks, artichokes—anything that has complex fiber and complex carbohydrates is an excellent prebiotic.

Even if you've taken a course of antibiotics, which can be harmful to gut bacteria, it's unlikely that you'll need to start taking probiotics—most of the time, an influx of prebiotics will help the body regain its natural balance.

In the vast majority of cases, a healthy, well-balanced, plant-based diet will provide everything you need. But if you have a condition that may necessitate probiotics, take it under the supervision of a gastroenterologist.

THE PROBLEM WITH EGGS

Although the relationship between egg consumption and blood cholesterol levels is not as clear as previously reported, there's good evidence that egg consumption increases the risk of cardiovascular disease and diabetes, which leads to cognitive decline. To our knowledge, no reliable data suggest that there is any benefit from eating more eggs. So why would we consume a food that is not beneficial when instead we can eat foods for which we have mountains of evidence showing they can reduce the risk of cardiovascular and brain diseases?—that is, plants.

WHAT ABOUT CHOLINE? Choline is an essential nutrient that helps the body maintain cellular structure, and it is a fundamental element of acetylcholine, which among its many roles in the body functions as a neurotransmitter. Humans produce choline in the liver, but the amount one

---

Gut-Brain Connection

There is an immense relationship between the gastrointestinal (GI) system and the nervous system. The vagus nerve, one of the most powerful parasympathetic nerves, is directly connected to the GI system, and your entire neural network interacts with your GI system in a way that is far more complex than simple digestion. What you eat has a direct and immediate impact on your brain, particularly when it comes to anxiety and depression.

The purpose of the parasympathetic nervous system is to calm the body, working to offset your limbic system, which, along with the sympathetic nervous system, tends to make the body more stressed. Because of its connection to the parasympathetic nervous system, your GI system controls your mood, which then controls your relationship with your sympathetic nervous system. You can calm your brain with the foods you choose to eat.

can synthesize is not quite enough to meet our needs. So we do need to get some in our diet, and egg yolk is high in choline.

True choline deficiency has been associated with Alzheimer's disease, cardiovascular diseases, liver disease, neuromuscular damage, and neural tube defects in newborns. But the science is not clear on how much choline we need, and this is where it gets murky. We actually don't have an established recommended daily intake. The data showing we need high amounts of choline come from a study conducted on only sixteen people about two decades ago.[8] But even most omnivores do not get the recommended level of choline suggested in that article.

Choline intake was a nonissue until 2019 when it was highlighted in an article authored by a UK nutritionist, who was on the board of the Meat Advisory Panel, who stated that vegans are choline-deficient.[9] She based her opinions on flawed and dated research on very sick people with low choline levels, who usually tend to have low levels of several critical micronutrients. There is absolutely no evidence that people who eat a plant-based diet have true choline deficiency. On the contrary, they have lower risk of Alzheimer's, stroke, and other cognitive diseases.

Regardless of conflicting opinions about choline intake, make sure you are consuming foods relatively high in choline until we have more evidence about what levels are safe and necessary. Yes, eggs contain choline, but so do many plant-based sources. Quinoa is high in choline, as are Brussels sprouts and chickpeas, which do none of the harm that eggs do *and* give you plenty of other benefits, besides.

In fact, there is actually evidence that we may be getting too much choline from meat and eggs, which leads to the formation of TMAO. As mentioned earlier, TMAO is associated with Alzheimer's and cardiovascular disease, among other diseases.

DIETARY CHOLESTEROL

Saturated fat is made out to be a villain of the standard American diet, and it should be. It is a nonessential nutrient, and its consumption has been associated with higher risk for Alzheimer's disease and cerebrovascular diseases. Cholesterol is an essential structural component of all cells, particularly brain cells. But our body produces enough cholesterol on its own, and the surplus is what contributes to vascular and neurodegenerative diseases. In a healthy brain, saturated fats and cholesterol can't get to the brain due to the presence of the tight junctions of the blood brain barrier, and any damage to this barrier increases the passage of LDL and cholesterol into the brain, causing damage to the neurons and other structures. Autopsy studies have found that brains of patients with Alzheimer's contained significantly more cholesterol than normal brains, and research conducted by Kaiser Permanente Northern California researchers found that individuals with high cholesterol levels during midlife had a 57 percent greater chance of developing Alzheimer's disease.[10]

There are several types of cholesterol. The two you're probably familiar with are low-density lipoprotein cholesterol (LDL, the "bad" cholesterol) and high-density lipoprotein cholesterol (HDL, the "good" cholesterol). LDL can damage your arteries and harden them, a process called atherosclerosis. Your heart therefore has to work much harder. Sometimes these plaques burst and form large clots that clog distal arteries, resulting in strokes and heart attacks.

But the problem isn't just atherosclerosis or vascular congestion—although these are bad enough. It's that there is evidence that LDL can cross the blood-brain barrier, and once it's in the brain it can undergo a process called auto-oxidation, which causes the formation of highly toxic free radicals. HDL, on the other hand, helps to clear such blockages, which is why there is a strong relationship between high HDL levels and greater health.

A diet rich in saturated fat increases the total cholesterol in the body (LDL and HDL). If you stop consuming saturated fats by switching to a plant-based diet, your total cholesterol will go down, including both LDL and HDL. Yes, your HDL levels may drop, but that isn't a bad thing. HDL is considered "good" because it reduces bad cholesterol deposition in the peripheral tissues by transferring it to the liver, where it is broken down. But as you improve your diet, you simply won't need it anymore. This is your body's way of balancing itself—it no longer needs as much HDL to combat a negative nutritional environment. If you see your HDL levels drop, it is probably congruent with a drop in LDL, which may be a good thing, because it means that your body is no longer in damage-control mode.

The key point here is that a low cholesterol level is good. Period.

THE DEAL WITH FAT: UNSATURATED FATS

All the data, from all the articles, research studies, clinical trials, and population studies, say that people who switch from animal-based diets to plant-based diets do extremely well. They are healthier overall, and they significantly reduce their risk of developing Alzheimer's and other forms of cognitive degeneration.

That said, the fact is that there are certain fats that are essential for brain health. We talked about how the brain is mostly made up of fat, and that's true—it has a proportionally higher amount of fat than most other organs. But that's all structural fat, the kind of fat our bodies can make on their own. The only fats the brain truly needs to get from our diet are omega-3s, which, as mentioned, can be easily found in marine algae, nuts, and seeds. Now, each of those contain other kinds of fats as well. Avocados, for instance, contain a lot of monounsaturated fat, but also some saturated fat, which is supposed to be bad, right?

So what's the answer? Eat fat or don't eat fat?

The answer is, it depends. If you are a healthy person with a good body mass index, a little extra virgin olive oil dressing on your salad isn't going to hurt you; in fact, it will probably help you. If you exercise and sleep well and are relatively stress-free, ditching the nutritious and delicious factor that makes it more likely that you're going to eat vegetables would just be silly. You don't need to eliminate unsaturated fats.

But if you're overweight, consuming calorie-dense foods like olive oil may not be helpful. Let's say we're talking about a man who is fifty years old, is overweight, and is prediabetic. In this case, we would want him to stay away from a lot of high-fat foods like oils, and increase consumption of a variety of unprocessed or minimally processed plants for a month, to help lose weight, and then slowly ease him back into consuming the healthier unsaturated fats, but in small amounts and as his health dictates. We are not against the consumption of cold-pressed extra virgin olive oil (EVOO), as plenty of research about the Mediterranean diet and patterns in the Blue Zones and from clinical trials has shown that its regular consumption is associated with a lower incidence of cardiovascular disease and cognitive decline. EVOO contains monounsaturated fats, phenolic compounds that are healthful for arteries, and other antioxidants. However, there are no data showing that an unprocessed plant–based diet with EVOO is superior to one without EVOO. Therefore, we feel that a diet can be healthy with or without the EVOO, depending on a person's baseline metabolic state. One thing is unequivocal: saturated fats and trans fats are harmful. In our recipes, we chose avocado oil as well, which has a similar profile as EVOO, because of its high smoke point compared with olive oil, so it's better for recipes requiring high-heat cooking.

BUT WHAT ABOUT KETO? The Ketogenic diet was discovered back in the 1920s to treat a small subtype of a rare childhood epilepsy intractable to medical treatment. Sure, ketogenic diet has been shown to have some very short-term positive effects for cognitive decline in a very small sample of people. But no data suggest that it is effective long term; in fact, there is evidence that it could be harmful especially when ketosis is achieved via the consumption of saturated fats. When you're eating too much saturated fats, it can lead to microvascular disease, which has been associated with Alzheimer's disease, not to mention the generation of inflammatory and oxidative by-products from high saturated fat consumption. In the absence of strong data supporting a ketogenic diet so far, and the presence of enough data

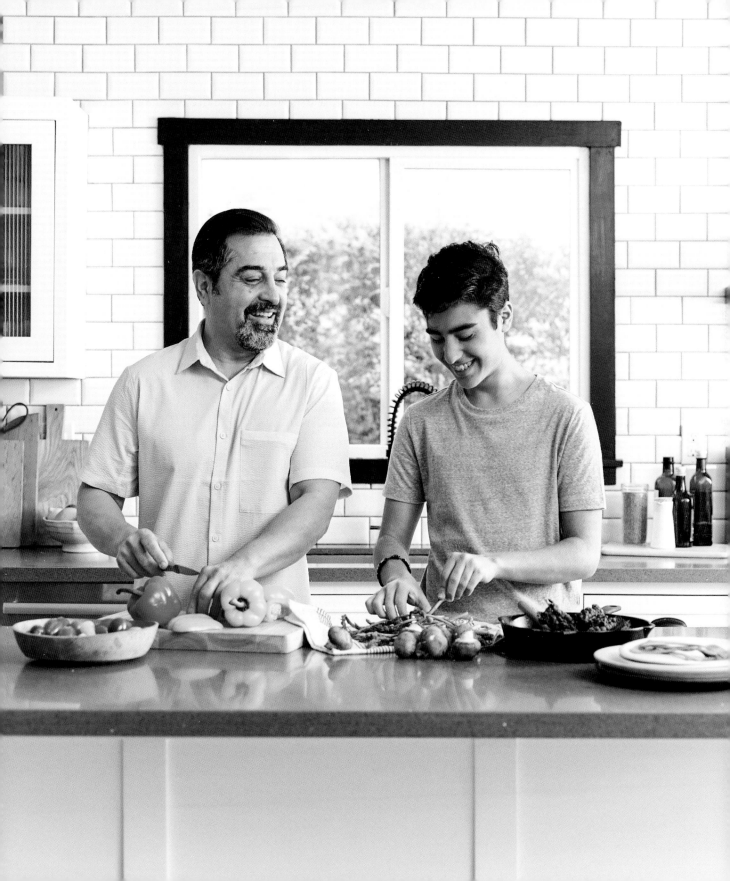

that shows the benefits of a plant-based diet, we do not recommend it—at least not through consumption of saturated fats.

The same applies to MCT oil, which stands for medium-chain triglycerides. MCT oil, as a product, is a manufactured form of saturated fat that's made by processing palm oil or coconut oil through a process called fractionation. Research is limited and has shown that MCT oil can help boost ketone production slightly. But so far there just isn't enough research on its benefits to show that it has a significant impact on brain function, and there is some indication that it might even worsen your cardiovascular health. Besides, for processed foods of any kind that don't have long-term studies, a healthy dose of skepticism is always a good idea.

AND WHAT ABOUT COCONUT OIL? Coconut oil is a rare plant oil that contains saturated fat—the other is palm oil. Coconut oil, however, has become something of a health celebrity for reasons we don't entirely understand. There have been some anecdotes about the ability of coconut oil to slow the progression of Alzheimer's, but this has never been verified in legitimate scientific studies. Coconut oil is about 90 percent saturated fat, which is a higher percentage than butter (about 64 percent saturated fat), beef fat (40 percent), or even lard (also 40 percent). Saturated fat increases cholesterol and consequently leads to an increased risk of dementia

and stroke and should therefore be avoided for better brain health.

THE THOUGHTFUL TWENTY BRAIN-NOURISHING FOODS

We just threw a lot of information at you. But we want you to know that the NEURO Plan is not that complicated. So what are the actual take-aways? What do you need to do to get started?

What follows are the Thoughtful Twenty brain-nourishing foods. While we believe dietary patterns, and not rigid food lists, are most beneficial for lasting brain health, we also understand that a list of specific foods is helpful for getting started. The NEURO 9 mentioned in Part 1 of this book are the essential foods that you must have every day while you are on the NEURO Plan. If you don't like broccoli, for example, you'll need to find another vegetable in the "crucifers" category of the NEURO 9 to fill that void. The Thoughtful Twenty listed below are an expanded list of foods that should be part of your brain-healthy menu, and will build out the foundations of your diet on the NEURO Plan.

1. LEAFY GREENS. These include kale, watercress, spinach, Swiss chard, collard greens, and arugula. Greens contain a ton of antioxidants, folic acid, vitamin E, and beta-carotene, all nutrients that support brain health.

2. **BROCCOLI.** Broccoli contains a special kind of antioxidant called Sulforaphane that can cross the blood-brain barrier and actually reverse damage caused by free radicals, and even normal aging.

3. **BLUEBERRIES.** In the anti-inflammatory index of foods, blueberries stand tall even in such good company as blackberries and strawberries. Their relation to the prevention of dementia has been studied extensively. They contain more polyphenolic compounds, specifically anthocyanins, which have anti-inflammatory and antioxidant effects. Anthocyanins have also been associated with increased neuronal signaling in areas of the brain that are responsible for memory function, and they improve the delivery of glucose to the brain. Studies have shown that when people regularly consume blueberries, they experience improved learning, better recall, and reduced symptoms of depression.

4. **MUSHROOMS.** Mushrooms improve overall immunity and contain polyphenols, which are natural antioxidants that prevent cellular damage. They are a great source of B vitamins such as B_2, niacin, and folate, which have all been shown to lower the risk of developing Alzheimer's.

5. **BEETS.** Beets contain folate, manganese, and copper, which are essential for maintaining neural infrastructure. They also contain compounds that create nitric oxide, which relaxes blood vessels, allowing more blood flow.

6. **AVOCADOS.** Avocados are packed with "good" fats, that is, monounsaturated fats that support brain structure.

7. **OLIVES.** Olives are a great source of polyunsaturated and monounsaturated fats. Unfortunately, most olives that we consume are dipped in a lot of salt water, but if you can find olives with a lower sodium content, they're great for you.

8. **NUTS, ESPECIALLY WALNUTS.** Although all nuts are good for you, walnuts are the best when it comes to brain health. They have relatively high amounts of omega-3 fatty acids in the form of ALA, as well as fiber and minerals. Walnuts have the highest antioxidants among nuts and can prevent LDL cholesterol–induced atherosclerosis. But don't go nuts with your nuts, for they are very high in calories. You don't want to eat a cup of walnuts a day; limit yourself to a quarter cup (or a handful). It's fine to eat nut butters as long as they are minimally processed—check the ingredients and make sure a nut butter is just nuts and doesn't contain added palm oil! Similarly, nut milks are great, but check to make sure you're not getting artificial ingredients or added sugar.

9. SEEDS. Flaxseeds, chia seeds, and sunflower seeds are loaded with nutrients. They are high in omega-3 fatty acids, protein, fiber, and minerals such as B vitamins, iron, and magnesium. The omega-3 fats are in the form of ALA, which as you recall converts to EPA and DHA, and provide sustenance to neurons. Flaxseeds also have lignans, which have antioxidant properties and fight degenerative changes in the body and brain.

10. BEANS AND LEGUMES. Beans contain resistant starches, fiber, plant proteins, antioxidants, phytonutrients, iron, and other minerals. They lower cholesterol and regulate blood sugar, and they also have been shown to increase longevity and reduce the risk of stroke.

11. QUINOA. Quinoa is incredibly rich in nutrients. It's the only seed that is a complete protein source, as many grains and seeds lack certain amino acids. It also contains fiber, vitamin E, zinc, phosphorus, and selenium, all essential for brain health.

12. OATS. Oats serve as a prebiotic and are an amazing source of a soluble fiber called beta-glucan. Beta-glucan reduces your bad cholesterol, feeds your good bacteria, and increases the feeling of fullness, so you're satiated with the smallest amount of oats, making weight loss easier. Oats also contain an

> ### What Is Amyloid?
>
> Amyloid is a by-product of a normal transmembrane protein, amyloid precursor protein, contained in most cells of the body, and every brain cell. Half of the amyloid precursor protein is contained within the cell, and the other half sticks out of it. When the body is under stress, this protein gets cut in the wrong place, and all those bits outside the cell begin to clump and tangle together. These are called beta-amyloid proteins, or amyloid for short. The body then attacks the amyloid, and when there is too much to handle, the immune system becomes overwhelmed, which becomes the beginnings of a destructive cascade.

exclusive form of antioxidant called avenanthramides. These antioxidants produce nitric oxide, which helps to lower blood pressure and increase blood flow to the small arteries of the brain. We enjoy our daily oatmeal with lots of toppings—berries, banana slices, walnuts, almond butter, flaxseeds, and chia seeds.

13. GREEN TEA. Green tea contains catechin, another polyphenol that activates toxin-clearing enzymes. It serves as a potent

anti-inflammatory. Recent research shows that consuming 1 to 2 cups of green tea a day lowers your risk of Alzheimer's and stroke because green tea contains the flavonoid compound EGCG (epigallocatechin gallate). EGCG crosses the blood-brain barrier and potentially prevents the aggregation of amyloid in the brain.

14. **TURMERIC AND OTHER SPICES.** Curcumin, found in turmeric, is an antioxidant, anti-inflammatory, and antiamyloid powerhouse. It has been shown to have a direct effect in reducing amyloid. It also has antibacterial properties, which is a nice bonus. We recommend that you eat at least half a teaspoon of turmeric per day. Adding a pinch of black pepper to turmeric increases its bioavailability by 2,000 percent. Spices are hands down the most anti-inflammatory food you can consume. The anti-inflammatory capacity of a quarter teaspoon of cloves is equal to *2 cups* of kale.

15. **CACAO.** Dark, unprocessed cocoa powder or cacao nibs are incredible sources of flavanol phytonutrients, which have been shown to relax arteries, allowing oxygen and other nutrients to reach the brain more easily. Cacao is a berry. The bitterness of cocoa is what makes it beneficial, so don't go out and eat a chocolate bar with all that added sugar and fat. Instead, add cocoa powder to your food, treating it like a spice.

16. **HERBS.** Cilantro, dill, rosemary, thyme, oregano, basil, mint, and parsley each contain ten times the antioxidants of nuts and berries. Spices contain the highest amounts of antioxidants per ounce compared with any other food and are excellent at supporting the brain's innate detox systems. Both spices and herbs like marjoram, allspice, saffron, nutmeg, tarragon, and others should be a regular part of your diet, not just a once-in-a-while addition.

17. **SWEET POTATOES.** Like legumes, sweet potatoes are packed with phytonutrients, fiber, vitamins A and C, minerals and fiber that can regulate your blood sugar.

18. **SOY.** There has been so much data on soy showing that it is beneficial in a variety of ways. Soy contains isoflavones, which have antioxidant and anti-inflammatory properties. It also has the highest content of protein in any legume and is high in iron and fiber. It has been shown to lower rates of cardiovascular disease by reducing total and LDL cholesterol, which in turn means better neurovascular function. The isoflavone is a type of phytoestrogen that does not mimic human estrogen, and in fact has been associated with

reduced risk of breast cancer and prostate cancer. Most dietary estrogen comes from meat and dairy products. Soy milk is great, as long as it doesn't contain added sugars. Consuming tofu, tempeh, and soy milk are great options for boosting your clean protein intake.

19. BRUSSELS SPROUTS. Brussels sprouts are high in fiber and contain a variety of vitamins, minerals, and antioxidants. They reduce inflammation, improve blood sugar control, lower cholesterol, and provide an immune boost—all of which benefit the brain. They are also incredibly low in calories; half a cup of Brussels sprouts contains only 25 calories.

20. GOJI BERRIES. This fruit is available dried, and it is an extremely effective anti-inflammatory. High in vitamins, goji berries also contain an antioxidant compound called zeaxanthin, which helps to regulate blood sugar and has been shown to improve sleep and reduce anxiety and depression.

FOODS TO AVOID

We went over much of this in Part 1, and all of this information is basically covered under our seven rules presented in Part 1, but we want to reemphasize and call out a few foods that you should absolutely refrain from eating during the thirty days of the NEURO Plan (and afterward, too!).

PROCESSED FOODS. Processed foods are high in salt, sugar, trans and saturated fats that damage the brain's arteries and tissue. This category includes meat substitutes and eggless mayo. It also includes white bread, white rice, white flour, and any other form of refined carbohydrates. The goal is to stick to one-ingredient foods during the month.

PROCESSED MEATS. Sandwich meat, salami, hot dogs, and bacon are all filled with salt, preservatives, and carcinogens and contain high amounts of saturated fat. They are packed with nitrosamines, a class of N-nitroso compounds—the same sort of stuff you find in cigarette smoke. N-nitroso compounds spontaneously decompose or are metabolized into highly reactive agents that are toxic to the brain. Processing meat by smoking or direct fire–drying often adds to the amount of nitrosamines it contains.

RED MEAT. Red meat is high in saturated fats and compounds such as AGEs, insulin-like growth factor 1 (IGF-1), and other reactive compounds. They also have high levels of nitrosamines, as well as heme iron, which is itself a pro-oxidant.

CHICKEN. Despite being purported as the "good" white meat, chicken is one of the main sources of saturated fats and AGEs in the standard American diet, simply because we eat so much of it. It can increase cholesterol levels at the same rate as beef.

BUTTER AND MARGARINE. These are both high in either saturated or trans fats, each of which can cause inflammation and damage arteries. More than that, these fats involve cellular processes that lead to cumulative waste, which can lead to significant vascular disease in the brain.

STORE-BOUGHT SALAD DRESSING. The vast majority of store-bought salad dressings are flat-out terrible for you, containing way too much sugar and salt and poor-quality fats. We provide recipes for making your own healthy salad dressings.

FRIED FOOD AND FAST FOOD. These foods are high in trans fats that damage brain arteries and other cellular structures of the brain, especially cell walls, leading to the progressive destruction of neurons and their supporting systems. Fried foods and fast foods contribute to cognitive decline and also tend to contain large amounts of salt, sugar, and preservatives—all bad for brain health.

CHEESE. Cheese is high in saturated fat, which damages blood vessels in the brain.

PASTRIES AND SWEETS. Needless to say, pastries and sweets are high in sugar, refined carbohydrates, and unhealthy fats—the combination of which can cause inflammation and brain burnout.

SWEETENED CHOCOLATE BARS. Don't be fooled by the word "chocolate." So often it is called a health food, but the reality is that in order for chocolate to have any health benefits, it needs to be free of sugar and contain a minimum 70 percent cacao. We're asking that you avoid sugar entirely during the thirty days of the NEURO Plan, but good-quality unsweetened cocoa powder is incredibly healthful, and if you want to use it, go for it!

SUGARY DRINKS. The main source of sugar in the standard American diet, sugary drinks cause inflammation, oxidation, and other cellular damage. Don't be fooled by juices and blended fruit mixes—these have stripped their fruits of their fiber and many of their nutrients, leaving behind nothing but sugar water.

ALCOHOL. Alcohol by nature is neurotoxic and directly damages brain cells, especially the connections between neurons. It can also negatively affect the gut microbiome, lowering the number of healthful bacteria. Some data show that drinking one glass of wine a day may have some benefit; however, we are learning that this benefit is not necessarily from the alcohol itself but from the convivial experience and relaxation that come with that glass of wine. Our advice is, if you don't drink alcohol, don't start. But if you do, keep to no more than a couple of glasses of wine a week in social settings, as anything more than that can damage your brain, both through its direct effects and through alcohol's negative impact on restorative sleep.

REFINED OILS. Refined tropical oils, such as coconut and palm oils, are high in saturated fatty acids and could increase inflammation. They also are high in calories and have no other nutrients at all. Extra virgin olive oil has been associated with a reduced risk of cardiovascular disease and Alzheimer's. It does not necessarily *have* to be a part of a healthy plant-based diet, but if you want to consume it in small amounts, it won't be harmful.

WHAT MAKES GREENS SO SPECIAL?

When you want more bang for your nutritional buck, eat your greens. Greens are one of the most nutrient-dense foods in the world; that is, they are high in nutrients and low in calories. They pack so much in: phytonutrients, vitamins, minerals, fibers, good carbohydrates, even proteins. Almost all studies done on brain health and nutrition, looking at either dietary pattern or factor analysis, show that the foods that stand out for people who have the best brain health and general health are greens. It's always greens.

On top of the greens list are kale and watercress. Kale has all of the good things listed above

plus omega-3 fatty acids. It contains compounds that feed your gut bacteria, which then help to produce short-chain fatty acids. A cup of kale provides 120 milligrams of omega-3s. Watercress is high in sulforaphane, a potent antioxidant compound.

> We have the power to make this life the best it can be. All it took was a book, and a doable plan. Every small step that I take moves me forward toward a future life that I can love and appreciate. Thanks for creating this program and sharing it for the good of all beings.
>
> —JOHN K.

WHAT ABOUT FRUIT AND OTHER "SWEET" WHOLE FOODS?

After what we've told you about processed sugar (and it really is terrible), you might be tempted to avoid sugar altogether, in all forms, and stop eating fruit or other sweet whole foods such as beets. But this isn't necessary. In fact, it's a bad idea.

Remember, the brain needs energy to run, and its preferred type of energy is glucose. Now, we're not taking back what we've said about sugar, so don't go out and eat a candy bar. Because while the brain does need that glucose, it needs to be delivered in a very specific way, with very specific timing. Your brain doesn't want a buffet; it wants a fancy sit-down dinner with four courses.

If your cells do not receive their glucose in appropriate increments, with an appropriate amount of time between, they will get overwhelmed. Fast sources of energy like processed sugar or ketones may give you a boost at first, but they will eventually cause inflammation, oxidation, and long-term damage. Too much sugar too rapidly can contribute to insulin resistance. Your insulin levels go up, but your cells can't recognize it until you're drowning in sugar your cells can't use.

It's like the difference between gasoline and nitromethane. Try running a Ford Pinto on nitro continuously for several years. That engine will burn out.

On the other hand, slow-releasing sources of glucose like whole fruits give your brain appropriate amounts of energy. When sugar is bound to fiber in a complex form, it has to be broken down, which allows it to be released slowly, in amounts that allow the body to absorb it, so the cellular system is not overwhelmed.

When people with poor insulin sensitivity and poor glucose tolerance eat a banana, they will experience an immense rise in their glucose level. And oftentimes they think, "The banana did this. It's all the banana's fault." But that's sim-

ply not true. If your glucose tolerance and insulin sensitivity have been damaged over the years by overconsumption of refined carbohydrates and saturated fats, then you will have a reaction to even healthy sugars like a banana. But as you cut out those refined sugars and bad fats, your sensitivity will return to normal. Whole fruits come packaged with water, fiber, antioxidants, vitamins, and minerals, and each of these serve as protective agents against blood glucose spikes and actually increase your sensitivity to insulin. Some fruits are naturally higher in sugar (mangoes and grapes), while others have less sugar (berries and stone fruits). If you're trying to get your insulin sensitivity back to normal, start off with low-sugar fruits and work from there.

NATURAL SUGARS. Yes, agave, molasses, honey, and maple syrup are relatively unprocessed when compared with refined sugar, but they lead to a glucose spike in the brain. They may be natural, but that doesn't mean they're good for you—in fact, they're quite the opposite.

CARBOHYDRATES ARE GOOD NOW?

Your brain runs on glucose. It is the only source of energy for the brain, unlike the rest of the body cells, which can use fats and proteins as fuels. There are really only three sources of macronutrients: proteins, fats, and carbohydrates. Let's look at them one at a time.

Proteins are not an efficient source of energy because they don't transfer well through metabolic processes, and in excess they can be toxic to the liver and kidneys. We need them, but our bodies can't run on them. Fats are high-energy molecules; they create twice as much energy as anything else. But of course, with such high energy, there are downsides. Saturated fats cause oxidation, and we aren't able to break them down completely. Ideally, our food is broken down to water, carbon dioxide, and adenosine triphosphate (ATP), the body's energy source. But fats can't get there; they get broken down only to ketones. In order to keep the energy-hungry brain going, ketones serve as a fuel when the body is under tremendous stress, such as during calorie restriction. Ketones are not the preferred source of energy for the brain; they are an emergency mechanism for brain survival. So ketones provide energy to cells, which is useful for short-term survival mode during times of starvation or for fight-or-flight mode, like running away from danger. But over the long term, ketones create oxidized by-products that eventually age the cells. Fats are quick, but in the absence of carbohydrates, they can be inefficient and harmful in the long run, as high-fat foods lack the vitamins and fiber that are crucial to keep the brain healthy.

We are left with carbohydrates. They are broken down efficiently into glucose, and they make it all the way to the final products of water, carbon dioxide, and ATP (the cell's optimal source of energy), allowing our cells to recognize and use this energy. This glucose easily crosses the blood-brain barrier to the brain cells. While the rest of the body cells can use fat and protein as fuel, the brain exclusively relies on glucose for fuel, which it needs constantly. And where does it come from? Our food.

Now, carbohydrates have developed a pretty bad reputation, because "good" and "bad" carbohydrates are not defined properly. There are many different types of carbs, and fiber is one of them. But for simplicity, we can separate them into simple (refined) carbs, which enter into your circulation quickly, and complex (unrefined) carbs, which require more digestion and provide a time-released energy. Lumping them together just doesn't work because you risk throwing the baby out with the bathwater. The carbs found in quinoa are very different from those found in boxed sugary cereal. The carbs in beans are very different from those in white pasta. The carbs in apples are very different from the sugar in soft drinks. The carbs in sweet potatoes are a world apart from the carbs in bagged chips.

Yes, Americans eat a lot of carbohydrates, but they are mainly coming from *refined* carbs in donuts, chips, pizza dough, white rice, condiments, pastries, and pasta. We're not getting them from *unrefined* carbs in oatmeal, quinoa, brown rice, sweet potatoes, berries, and other plants. And that's the difference. We completely agree with cutting out refined carbs like white flour and various processed carbs like crackers and chips. But do whole grains really need to go? Absolutely not. Carbohydrates are too important for proper brain function.

Carbohydrate-restricting diets have been around for a long time, and typically they place carbohydrate intake at less than 50 grams daily. But the research into such diets is quite limited at the population level. One of the few populations studied that had a low-carbohydrate, high-fat and high-protein diet were the Inuits. Their diet wasn't really one we can achieve these days (not many opportunities or much desire to eat seal or whale meat), and we wouldn't really want to: the Inuit population studied did not have exceptional health or longevity, and they were actually subject to higher incidents of intracranial hemorrhage and cardiovascular disease at a younger age, likely because of their high fat consumption.[11]

On the other hand, when we look at Blue Zone populations—like the Okinawans in Japan, the Seventh-Day Adventists in Loma Linda, the Ikarians in Greece, and the Sardinians in Italy—we find that each of them eats a diet high in whole grains, including breads—but not the kinds of breads you usually see in the grocery store. These breads are made with 100 percent stone-ground whole wheat, as close to the natural unprocessed form of wheat as possible.

It is true that a low-carb diet may help you lose weight. But with all the saturated fats and protein you're replacing it with, you're losing the brain-preserving qualities of resistant starches and fiber; you're increasing inflammation in the brain; and you're increasing your risk for high blood pressure, high cholesterol, and insulin resistance—each of which can lead to massive brain damage in the form of strokes and/or dementia.

Again, there are good carbs and there are bad carbs. The problem with carbohydrates is that we have messed with them, that is, processed them, making them less complex and taking away the fiber and other nutrients that allow the body to absorb and use them. So we're definitely not telling you to eat donuts for brain health. But if you eat carbohydrates in whole form—including fruits, vegetables, whole grains, nuts and seeds, legumes, and more—your body can process all that good glucose it gets from them and present it to the brain in a controlled form.

BUT WHAT ABOUT GLUTEN? Gluten is a wheat protein. Only 1 to 2 percent of people are very sensitive to gluten, but it seems like *everybody's* giving up gluten these days. For about 90 percent of people, it is just as health-promoting as any other plant-based protein.

There are a few reasons people may have for avoiding gluten, in particular, celiac disease, but only one in one hundred people has this disease. Only one in a thousand people has a wheat allergy. Then there are gluten sensitivities, and it's difficult to say how common those are. Our best estimate at this point is that 1 percent of the population has celiac disease, 2 percent of the population is sensitive to gluten, and maybe another 1 to 2 percent is sensitive to wheat. Except in the case of celiac disease, these sensitivities can come at different levels, some so minor as to not be detected when eating a whole-food diet.

If you don't have celiac disease or wheat or gluten sensitivity, there is no reason why you shouldn't eat gluten. Americans' gluten concerns have been blown way out of proportion, and

> ### *Quinoa*
>
> **We're going to call out quinoa because, frankly, it's just amazing. It's called a pseudo grain because it is actually a seed. Just half a cup of quinoa has 4 grams of protein. It contains all nine essential amino acids, including the ones you can usually find only in animal products. You can definitely call quinoa a superfood (despite that word being tossed around so much these days). It's an anti-inflammatory, an antioxidant, and contains 25 grams of fiber per 1-cup serving. You're going to see a lot of quinoa in our recipes.**

we believe that many of the symptoms people are attributing to gluten likely come from processed foods. There is no evidence to suggest that following a gluten-free diet has any significant benefits for the general population. In fact, evidence suggests that a gluten-free diet may adversely affect your gut health, essentially working as an antibiotic, killing off the good bacteria in the gut. Data from the National Health and Nutrition Examination Survey suggests that whole-grain intake is related to positive nutrient profiles and lowers risk of chronic disease, including cancer, *and* it results in better control of body weight.[12]

Unless you have a good medical reason for it, there is no reason to go gluten-free. Certain population studies have found that dietary grains actually appear strongly protective in relation to Alzheimer's disease. In other words, perhaps don't pass on the grain—instead, pass the grain, to spare the brain.

WAIT, I CAN EAT BREAD? Yes, you absolutely can! Whole grains are *healthy*, not harmful, so yes, you can have a 100 percent whole-wheat bun with your veggie burger! You can have a slice of sourdough toast with nut butter. Enjoy!

WHAT ABOUT NIGHTSHADES?

The concerns over the nightshade family of foods, such as tomatoes, peppers, eggplants, and white potatoes, are similar to the concerns over gluten: a small number of people (even smaller

than those with gluten sensitivities) have an issue with them, and therefore must avoid them. The fact is, there is no evidence that nightshades are bad for the brain. Yes, some conditions can make nightshades bad for you, say, if you've got specific diagnosed rheumatological or autoimmunological diseases. In those cases, when you have a lot of inflammation, your body will have a difficult time digesting nightshades.

But bell peppers, tomatoes, eggplants—all of these pack a lot of good stuff in them! They are the cornerstone of the Mediterranean diet, which has been shown to offer a host of benefits, including weight loss, heart health, cancer prevention, diabetes prevention and control, and of course brain health. Once again, if you have issues with nightshades, then stay away from them, but if not, go ahead and reap the benefits of these healthy vegetables.

DO I NEED TO TAKE SUPPLEMENTS?

Some people believe that people following a plant-based diet are deficient in some vitamins and minerals and need to take supplements. Current data show, however, that if you are eating a well-rounded diet, you do not need vitamin supplements. In fact, if you take them when you don't need them, they can become problematic. Too much vitamin A can lead to blurred vision and bone pain, while too much vitamin D can cause nausea and headaches as well as heart, kidney, and respiratory issues. There is also evidence that an excess of certain vitamins may, over time, increase the risk of certain types of cancers. The reality is that biohacking in this way doesn't work. Maybe one day we will have the technology to create drugs that can supercharge our systems, but we're not there yet. In the meantime, you can get the micronutrients you need from a well-rounded, diverse, and unprocessed plant–based diet.

The only supplement that you will likely need is vitamin B_{12}, regardless of whether you are eating a plant-based diet, as omnivores are also deficient. If you eat a well-balanced and well-planned diet, you will not need any additional supplements. To be safe, the best thing to do is to get your vitamin and mineral levels checked once a year. If they're low, you should work with your physician to understand *why* they're low—because of diet? or because of some underlying medical problem? If you find no underlying cause for deficiency, then and only then should you turn to supplements.

OMEGA3. Taking an algae-based omega-3 supplement would ensure adequate DHA levels if you are not getting enough from plant-based sources.

BUT WHAT ABOUT IRON? In terms of supplementing the diet with vitamins and minerals, we hear a lot about iron. But a well-rounded plant-based diet not only has enough iron, it has the *right* kind of iron. Heme iron (the kind of iron found in meats) is toxic and has been shown to increase the risk of cancer, stroke, heart disease, and metabolic syndrome, whereas non-heme iron doesn't become the source of oxidized damage. It's true that heme iron is more readily absorbed than non-heme iron—and that's precisely why the amount absorbed by the body can continue to rise even if the body doesn't need any iron, and cause oxidative damage to the brain. Some studies indicate that excessive iron intake is associated with several neurodegenerative diseases such as Parkinson's and Alzheimer's disease.[13]

Non-heme iron is absorbed in a regulated way, such that the body takes it in only if it needs iron. If you avoid heme iron, over time your body will start to absorb non-heme iron more easily, especially if it's accompanied with foods high in vitamin C, such as bell peppers, tomatoes, broccoli, citrus fruits, strawberries, apricots, kiwi fruits, and pineapples. Great sources of plant-based iron are dark leafy greens like kale, beans, chia seeds, tofu, tempeh, and dried apricots.

CHALLENGES THAT WILL COME UP

When you change your diet from the standard American diet to an unprocessed plant–based one, issues will arise that you will have to deal with. But you *can* deal with them.

MY ENERGY LEVELS ARE DOWN. You often feel like you have less energy when you change your diet as we suggest. And, in fact, you *do* have less energy—at least at first. You're consuming fewer calories, because these new foods contain fewer calories, not to mention less sugar and fat. Your body is used to receiving a certain amount of sugar and a different type of fat (unhealthy fats), and it believes this is what it needs to function (but it's wrong about that). Think about eating a donut versus eating a salad: you'd have to eat truckloads of salad to feel the sugar and fat rush you get from a donut. You're depriving your body of its rush, and it's going to be angry at you about it for a while. In a way, your body is going to go through withdrawal for the first few days to a week of the new way of eating.

I'M STILL HUNGRY. We all know that lower calorie intake makes people healthier, but that doesn't mean it feels good right away. You're moving away from calorie-dense/nutrient-sparse foods; and while you're making that change, you'll sometimes feel hungry, as if your brain and body aren't getting the fuel they need. You *are* getting enough food, but remember that a donut has 400 to 700 calories, while a nice, big, nutrient-dense salad has only 300 calories. Your body knows it's getting less, and it's going to make sure you know it, too. So you won't feel satiated right away—but that will change, and faster than you think. In the meantime, eat foods that require a lot of chewing to help remind your body that you are in fact eating plenty of food. Eat healthy fats that help you feel full, including nuts and avocados. Eat beans and whole grains packed with plenty of protein, fiber, and complex and resistant starches that expand your stomach and make you feel full. We will help you eat at least 1,500 calories a day so you can make it through this, but hang in there through the withdrawal.

I DON'T FEEL GOOD. You might feel like you're getting a virus, like you just don't *feel good*. That happens, as your body is experiencing some discomfort as it learns to manage new input. You're asking your body to digest and convert all kinds of new foods in new quantities, and it's not getting any job training. There's going to be some dissonance. Your body is going to feel like something is wrong, since it's being asked to do things it doesn't usually have to do (like digest a whole lot of greens). Like most of us, when your body is asked to do new things, it rebels: "This is hard! I don't like it!" The good news is that your body is a fast learner, and it'll realize quickly enough that actually, it doesn't run all that well on Dunkin'.

I DON'T LIKE THE TASTE OF THIS FOOD. This is some healthy food you're eating, and a lot of us have a negative association with healthy food—we believe it tastes bad. But the truth is, taste isn't taste; taste is habit. All around the world, people enjoy foods that might make you nauseous, but they think those foods are delicious. (And conversely, they think some of the foods in the standard American diet are disgusting.) But we're all the same species, and we all have the same taste buds. We just have different customs, habits, history, culture, and availability of foods, and those things are what inform our interpretations of how things taste. Your sense of taste will change as your habits change. Your taste for most foods can adjust in fewer than two weeks, though some foods may take as long as a month. But you will get used to these new foods, and as you do, you will come to crave them, so much so that you will no longer be able to imagine going back to the standard American diet.

I REALLY CRAVE SUGAR. Ayesha was addicted to sugar. She still is, in fact. Sadly, this is one of those cravings that is never going to go away. To this day, if Ayesha sees a donut, she still wants to gobble it up—and it's been fifteen years since that was a part of her diet! Just like with any other addiction, with sugar, you're always a recovering addict. Your brain responds to it the same way it does to heroin, so cut yourself a little slack when you experience sugar cravings. They're normal. But remember what happens on the other side of that donut, and reach for one

of the replacements we offer to get you through the tough moments.

AND I CRAVE SALT, TOO. We promise you that we're not cutting out salt entirely, we're just minimizing it. We eat *so much salt* in the standard American diet, way more than food needs in order to taste good—but again, that's what we're used to. It'll take a little while for you to get used to smaller amounts of salt, both from a taste and cravings perspective, but you *will* get used to it. And you will eventually find that you enjoy being able to taste the flavors that were "underneath" the salt before—the natural flavors of so many foods, and the herbs and spices that are, pound for pound, the most anti-inflammatory and antioxidant compounds in existence.

I REALLY CRAVE CHEESE AS WELL. We provide swaps and foods that resemble the umami, or savory flavor, of cheese, but that salt/fat combo, plus the casomorphin factor, is going to make giving up cheese a bit of a rough ride at first. But you can do it. Hang in there!

WHAT ABOUT MEAT CRAVINGS? Ayesha swears that Dean was a wolf in a previous life. When she first met him, he kept only meat in his fridge. These cravings are real, but they will go away, especially if you make an effort to replace your meat protein with vegetable proteins, as we recommend.

HOW TO GET THROUGH THE THIRTY DAYS OF THE NEURO PLAN

All right, so it isn't going to be easy. But it's not impossible, and there are some things you can do to help your body get through these challenges. We think of this as nutritional jujitsu. In jujitsu, you take your opponent's force and energy and use it to your benefit. Here, we show you how to take the things that are harming you, like fat, sugar, and salt, and replace them with things that are not only not harmful but are actively *good* for you. If you feel any cravings, try one of these swaps instead.

SUGAR. It's possible to get the sweetness of sugar without the harmful effects. First of all, we're not against artificial sweeteners. Monk fruit extract is our preference, but as far as brain health is concerned, there is no clear evidence that erythritol causes any problems. There have been some anecdotes about stevia causing brain fog, and since there hasn't been any research into its safety, we're not comfortable saying it's safe. But if you're going to use any kind of artificial sweetener, don't consume a truckload of it. Do what feels right for you, and be wise about it. Monk fruit extract is the most natural form of sweetener out there. It has just a few calories per serving.

SALT. First of all, we're not asking you to give up salt entirely. A small amount of salt used as a flavor-enhancer is fine, but anything more than a teaspoon a day is harmful. Unfortunately, you're probably used to high salt levels, and you'll need some support in cutting back. Replacing that excess salt with more herbs and spices will quickly help you realize that not only does your food taste better, but you feel better, too.

TEXTURE AND SAVORY FLAVORS OF MEAT. The chewy texture and umami flavors of meat can easily be found elsewhere. We will show you how to create amazing recipes with vegetables, whole grains, legumes, and a variety of herbs and spices so that your meals are packed with flavor and that savory chewiness you may be craving.

CHEESE. Eating nutritional yeast and nut cheeses (check out our recipe for Chipotle Cashew Queso! [page 205]) will satiate your cravings for cheese. You will notice how wonderful you feel without cheese very soon!

FATS. We aren't getting rid of all fats in your diet. But we are replacing them with good, healthy fat, like those in nuts or avocados or nut-based creams. Any cravings for bad fats will go away as your body adjusts to more healthy fats.

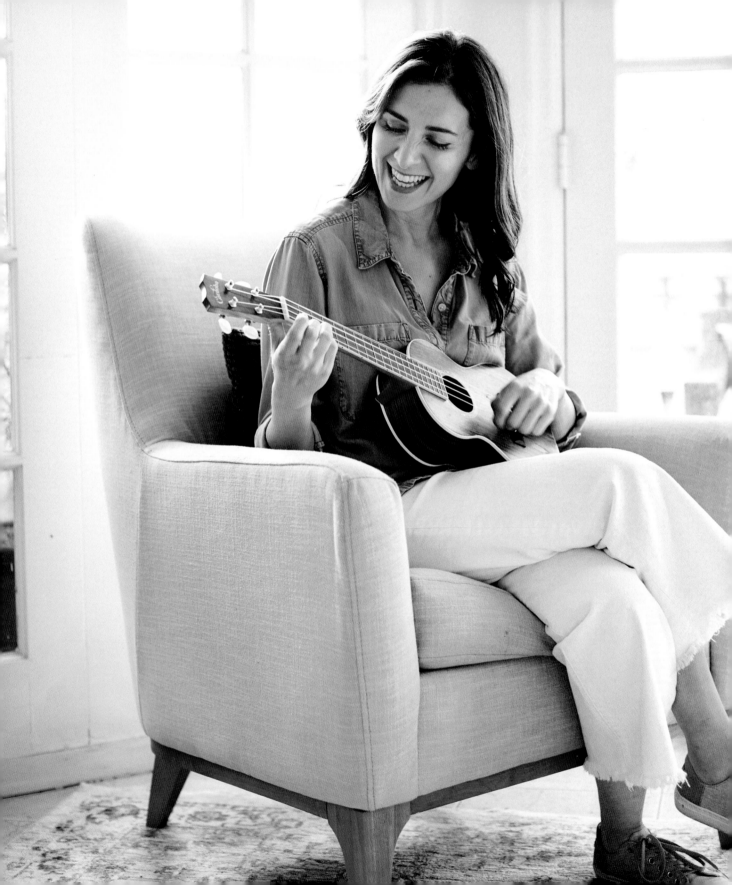

HOW TO SUCCEED AND HOW TO FAIL

Our work with the brain and behavior has helped us understand that we all take certain steps to build a habit. If you think about getting healthy being like climbing up a mountain—and it feels that way sometimes—then you know how you start at the bottom and just take one step at a time. But if you skip a step, it's easy to slip and fall.

So let's consider: Where are you on that mountain? Where are you on the journey of change? At the very bottom is PRE-CONTEMPLATION, when you're unaware of the *need* to change. If you're reading this book, you're likely well past this step, but it's helpful to look at *all* your behaviors as they concern the spectrum of NEURO—Nutrition, Exercise, Unwind, Restore, and Opti-

mize. Are there areas that perhaps you didn't realize needed work? Perhaps you didn't see how little sleep you get or how negatively stressed you are. Look at the whole picture.

Or you may be at the stage of CONTEMPLA-TION, when you are aware of the need for change and actively want to do so, but you haven't yet started. Again, if you've made it this far in the book, you're probably past this step, too—but a lot of folks just stay here, stuck, knowing they need to make a change but never doing anything about it.

In all likelihood, you're at the PREPARATION stage, when you're learning what you need to do in order to change. Simply the act of reading this book is an act of preparation.

But we can't stop there; that's only halfway up the mountain. We're going to walk with you from here, supporting you as you take the next step: ACTION. This is when you begin to practice distinct behaviors that will produce the desired changes—eating well, sleeping well, exercising, socializing, all the things you now know you need to do to be healthy.

You've probably been here before. You've probably been on diets, and it went great for a while . . . until it didn't. This is because you didn't take the next step, and it's likely the hardest one: MAINTAINING SUSTAINABLE BEHAV-IOR. You have to make a commitment for these thirty days of the NEURO Plan, and stick with it—through the thirty days and beyond for a lifetime of change.

We've noticed that, most often, making a commitment to maintaining sustainable behavior is the biggest challenge. It's not the change in diet; it's the decision to make that change. We see two things that get in the way of making this decision: MOTIVATION and MODERATION. Those words typically have a positive connotation, but, well, not to put too fine a point on it, we hate them.

First, let's talk about "motivation." This is our least favorite word, because it's essentially meaningless and it's impossible to hang on to. The subconscious brain is like a toddler. It understands two things: I like it, and I don't like it. Honestly, when you introduce your brain to a new diet, it's not going to like it. So there goes your motivation, immediately. Your brain, caught up in its comfortable limbic, habitual state, says, "No, thank you"; and then because your brain is not on board with this enormous change, you feel like a failure, and you give up.

We invite you to think about motivation in a different way—the way you think about love: love isn't a noun, it's a verb. It's something you *do*, all day, every day, forever, and it requires systematic effort on your part. The common understanding of motivation is that it's supposed to just be there for you, that it's a noun you can rely on; but that's simply not true. Motivation isn't something you *have*, it's something you *do*,

and it requires effort. True motivation is a process, and it builds over time. It starts with your purpose—and we don't mean anything grand, like your "life's work," but something you desire that will take some time to achieve.

It helps to have some tension here; make sure your purpose isn't too simple or easy to achieve. It has to be achievable, but it also needs to require some work. When you set clear goals that are driven by that purpose, you are creating a basis for true motivation. Every time you succeed at a goal, you create a pattern of behavior. Remember, your brain functions in a binary way: "I like it" and "I don't like it"—those are the only options. The more you succeed, the more your brain says "I like it," and so the more it works to succeed. Once this pattern is established, you have the driving force of motivation working for you.

Runner-up for our least favorite word is "moderation." We hear this all the time: "It's fine to eat meat—in moderation." "It's fine to eat sugar—in moderation." The problem is that everyone experiences "moderation" differently. Eating bad fats "in moderation" will mean something very different to someone who eats a cheeseburger every day and someone who has been plant-based for years. The unfortunate truth is that, according to the American Heart Association, only about 0.4 percent of Americans are eating a healthy diet, so the general concept of "moderation" likely skews heavily in one direction. If you are eating burgers and fries five times a day and you decrease your consumption to three times a day, that's eating in moderation for you; but that many burgers and fries is still going to make you very, very sick. It's like saying, "I consume poison only in moderation." How is that helpful? We argue for an approach that measures each person against optimal health, knowing that each step in the right direction yields results.

WHAT WORKS

We've talked a lot about what *doesn't* work—so what *does* work? How exactly do you make that commitment?

The first step is understanding *why* it's hard. The fact is that this is just how human beings are built, because like all animals, we're fixated on survival. And survival means what's happening *right now*, not what might happen one day in the future if we don't do something. "One day in the future" is just too vague a fear for a brain that's designed to fear scary, immediate instances like facing a predator in the wild. If you're hungry and grumpy, all your brain cares about is that feeling. You'll obey the urge to grab a donut, even though you know it's just going to make you hungrier and grumpier later. "Later" is somebody else's problem, according to your brain, and this inability to value "later" is why it's hard for us to form healthy habits. The immediate want and the immediate gain always stand in the way.

We're going to give the brain what it needs and thrives on: immediate gains that are relevant, measurable, and something to celebrate. Did you make it through the first of the thirty days of the NEURO Plan? Celebrate that! Track your progress on a whiteboard, and make sure you put it somewhere where you'll see it. Rather than trying to distract your brain from what you're doing, *focus* on it, in a positive way.

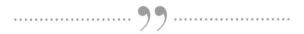

Here are some of the things that I have learned that I now do on a consistent basis. I've changed how I eat and I try to stick to mostly a plant-based way of eating. However, I do slip from time to time, but when I do, I instantly can feel the difference and I go back to a more plant-based way of eating. I am doing some form of exercise when I get home at night. I am still working on learning to meditate and have it be a norm for me. I've changed how I sleep at night, but I still need to work on getting in bed and getting up at the same time. I love to dance so incorporating that into my daily habits was the easiest thing that I could do for myself. And I learned to set an intention and actually keep it.

—SARAH, AGE THIRTY-FIVE

Yes, at first your brain won't like it. Your amygdala is addicted to sugar and bad fat, and just as if you were cutting out addictive drugs, your brain will yell at you, demanding that it receive its supply. Going back to sugar and bad fats because

of those demands will *feel* rewarding—just like going back to cocaine would feel good. But that doesn't mean it *is* good. Your brain needs some training to become addicted to something else: success, and the benefits of good food. You can and will become addicted to this success; your basal ganglia will literally change, and each day will get exponentially easier.

HOW TO BUILD POSITIVE HABITS

By their very nature, habits aren't something people tend to give a lot of thought to. We create them without even realizing it, without understanding how we got there—which of course is why when we say "habits," we generally mean "bad habits."

One of the things that makes the NEURO Plan different is that we are not only neurologists; we're neurobehavioral neurologists. Our work is centered on neurological and nutritional science *and* a well-established behavior modification program. We will help you take on habit-building in a proactive, intentional manner so that you can overcome the patterns laid down during your early years when your immediate physical needs, as well as any fears or insecurities, were the driving force of all your behavior. Comfort eating? That's a habit. Binge-watching TV? That's a habit. These habits were built when you were young and long-term planning was even more impossible for your brain to consider than it is now.

Let's look at how these habits could have been created. Imagine you're in high school and it's finals week. You haven't studied, because you've been busy with friends or sports or parties or any of the other things you did in high school (we won't ask). But then, oh man, it's the night before a final, and you stay up all night studying, scarfing down pizza and Red Bull or Mountain Dew or whatever other revolting caffeine-filled drink you think you need to get through the night. You don't fail, so you decide (consciously or unconsciously) that this was a successful tactic. So you do it again next term, and the term after that, through college and into your job today. Maybe you don't pull so many all-nighters, but you do procrastinate and you do "treat yourself" to highly processed snacks to get you through stressful days.

This is now a lifelong habit, and when you're in your forties, fifties, or later, and you're still living in urgency mode, those habits are very hard to break. Your brain prefers habit-driven behaviors because those behaviors don't require any work from the higher cortical brain, which needs lots of energy to operate. Habits are mostly laid down in the inner basal ganglia, which require less energy. Autopilot mode is much easier on the brain, but that doesn't mean it's good for it, or for you.

Now, it is difficult to get rid of habit-driven behaviors. Those pathways have been hardwired in your brain, and it takes a lot of work to transform those bad habits into good ones—like walking through deep snow to make a track. The first few times it will be hard as you feel all the resistance from the snow, but once you walk on that path multiple times and tamp down the snow, you'll be able to walk on it without any resistance.

It isn't easy, but it can be done. It requires two things: MINDFULNESS, a buzzword these days, but basically here meaning the act of consciously, intentionally, and proactively deciding on behaviors that serve your purpose; and a SYSTEMATIC, SUCCESS-BASED REPETITION, to lay down positive-habit pathways in the brain.

SET SMART GOALS

We are nerdy neurobehavioral neurologists, so of course we have to break it down. In order to intentionally create good habits, you have to have a plan for how you're going to get somewhere. And generally speaking, it takes some time. Seven days isn't long enough to form a habit. Two weeks isn't long enough to transform a habit. Based on our experience, thirty days is long enough to create a significant core set of fundamental habits upon which you can base the rest of life.

One step is action. Three steps form a pattern. Nine steps build a habit. Twenty steps create a behavior. And after that? It's character. This is now *who you are*. If we can teach you to identify your successes and continue to change, then our work is done, because that's all you need. It becomes a positive addiction.

The way to get this positive snowball effect started is to set some goals. But they can't be vague, long-term goals like "lose thirty pounds" or even "don't get Alzheimer's." Remember how your brain feels about long-term planning. Instead, you have to be SMART. Make sure your goals are:

S = SPECIFIC. Instead of the vague "be healthy," try "avoid adding refined sugar to my coffee for thirty days," or better yet, "follow the rules of the NEURO Plan for thirty days."

M = MEASURABLE. Your goals have to be quantifiable. "Eat more vegetables" is virtually meaningless, while "eat three servings of kale a week" is something you can measure and know you have achieved.

A = ATTAINABLE. If you can't succeed at your goal, it won't do you any good. Is "I will run a marathon at the end of these thirty days" possible if you've never jogged more than 5 miles in your life? Nope. That goal is not attainable. Try "I will jog 1 mile three times a week for a month."

R = RELEVANT. This is about setting goals that are connected to your higher purpose. If your higher purpose is ultimately achieving a whole-food, plant-based diet, then your goals should include eating meals for a week that are consistent with that higher purpose. If your higher purpose is to exercise one day for ninety minutes, then a ten-minute walk every day for a week will serve that higher purpose.

T = TIME BOUND. Each of the above examples has set a time limit. When your goals have no specific end time, you have no way of knowing whether you've achieved them. Now, it's true that our goal for you is to live a lifetime following the NEURO Plan, but these SMART goals are intended to help you build the habits that will make that possible. Set appropriate time limits for yourself, knowing that you will create new goals once you have achieved these.

When you've achieved a goal, take a moment to celebrate your success. This is extremely important, not just because you deserve it (although you do!) but because your brain needs to experience that success. In order to change your behavior and move past your habits, you have to do more than just repeat new behaviors. Your default system—your habits—is already in place, and it has been formed by repetition over so many years that it will take at least as many years to overcome it through repetition alone. There has to be a reward system that turns on the dopamine and lets your brain know that these changes actually *feel good*. You will become addicted to that dopamine rush, and that will be enough to change your habits.

So what's a good reward? Well, it shouldn't be food. If you treat yourself to a cupcake after a week of kale, all you're doing is digging into your old habits. Sure, overall you'll be healthier, but if you're trying to create new habits, that cupcake will only undo all the good work you've done. Instead, you'll create a kind of dysfunctional mindset, teaching your brain that the rest of your food is not pleasurable. You need to allow your brain to develop a taste for healthy foods.

Instead, choose a reward that is behavior-based. Celebrate by going on a hike with friends, taking a yoga class, or reading a good book. And if it just so happens that your reward helps you engage in some of the other aspects of the NEURO Plan, then all to the better!

Once you've taken the time to celebrate, it's critical to reassess and re-create new goals each time you complete one. Start thinking about this right away, because if you let some time elapse, it will be more difficult to keep building on your accomplishment. Create a SMART goal that is a next logical step from your previous success, so you can keep your momentum going.

How long will it take for these goals to turn into patterns and then to become habits and finally a way of life? We wish we could give you a concrete answer, but the reality is that everyone is different. These thirty days will get you going toward establishing a strong foundation—and for some of you, even a habit—but remember that it does take time beyond that. This is a kick-start, but when the thirty days are up, you will still have work to do. How long it will take beyond the thirty days depends on your history of habit-creating, on your previous level of self-discipline, and on all the other factors in your life, such as medical conditions, family demands, work demands, and so forth. But remember: no matter what those factors are—and no matter how overwhelming you believe them to be—this program works *every time*, even if it might take a little longer, as long as you stay consistent and maintain your goal-setting behavior.

These thirty days will allow you to create fundamental changes in your behaviors and habits, changes that you can build on for the rest of your life. This is a habit-creating period covering all aspects of the NEURO Plan, and once you've created these new, positive habits, changing your life becomes easy.

GREATER SUCCESS WITH A PARTNER

It helps to do this with a partner—though it isn't absolutely necessary. A NEURO partner can be a local friend, a friend across the country, a coach, a sister, a brother, a husband, a wife, a neighbor, or an online community like the one you can find through our website, teamsherzai.com.

One factor that contributes the most to long-term success is having a "tribe." For instance, Okinawa, one of the Blue Zones, has an interesting social aspect—people there tend to form cohorts, a group of five people aligned together from birth called *moai*. These five people go through their lives together, supporting and taking care of one another. These cohorts were found to contribute enormously to the longevity of the people of Okinawa.

Optimize, the fifth facet of the NEURO Plan, went into this in detail: a sense of community is key to mental and indeed all physical health. In our work, we promote working in groups much like the Okinawan cohorts that will go through their health journey together. This kind of cohort will help you, too.

By "cohort" we mean the small group of people, or even just one person, that you rely on the most. This is the person or people whom you confide in, whom you count on, whom you are there for when they need you, and who will always be there for you. When you look back, these people have helped shape your habits—and they can continue to do so. Your cohort can empower your healthy choices and hold you accountable for making them.

Now, it might be that this person is not at the same place in the journey as you are. Remember that mountain of change? Maybe you're at "action," but your tribe is still at "pre-contemplation." It would of course be most helpful if they were at the same stage as you and could do these thirty days with you, but it isn't absolutely necessary. What is necessary is making sure that your tribe supports you as you make this change. You cannot have the people you rely on sabotaging your efforts, saying things like, "Oh, one ice cream cone won't hurt!" or "Skip leg day at the gym today and come to the movies with me instead"—not when you've set a goal for yourself that you are trying so hard to accomplish successfully.

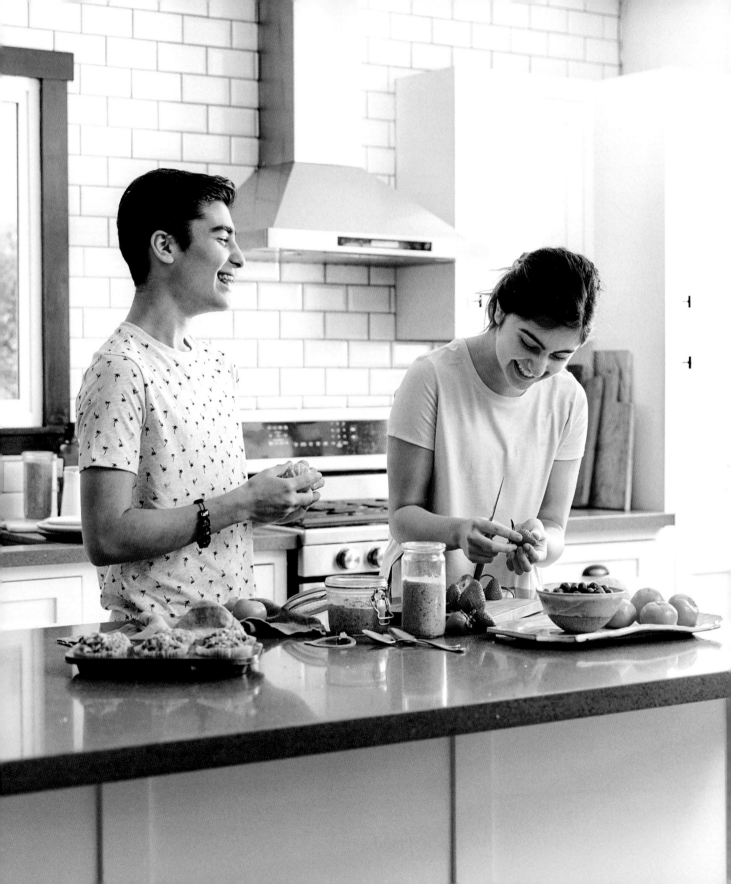

Consistently succeeding is critical to behavior change and habit formation, and consistent failure will create a habit of failure.

We know that many of you have partners at home who are not aligned with your changes. We get it, and we know it makes things harder. But your partner doesn't *have* to make the same changes you do; all that is necessary is that he or she supports you in your change. Before you begin, have a heart-to-heart conversation with your tribe and explain very clearly what you are going to do and why, and ask for their support. These people love you, and they will support you in this.

If someone in your tribe wants to join you, terrific! If not, find another partner or group to go along with you. Set goals together and make sure you keep each other accountable in an empowering and encouraging way. This kind of support can be pivotal for your success in long-term brain health.

TIPS AND TRICKS FOR DEALING WITH REALITY

A thirty-day overhaul of the way you eat, cook, and live isn't easy, particularly when life gets in the way. How do you eat healthy when you've got hungry kids who eat only chicken nuggets and pizza? Takeout is bad, but who has time to cook? How do you eat healthy when Jen from Accounting is always bringing donuts to the office? What do you do when someone offers you birthday cake and ice cream?

These are the real, everyday challenges that can send us tumbling back down that mountain—but they don't have to. Here are some simple strategies for dealing with these roadblocks:

COOK IT YOURSELF. Takeout *is* generally unhealthy. We offer lots of recipes in this book because—you guessed it—it's best to cook your food yourself. This isn't just for reasons of nutrition but because the time you spend making your own food can give you a greater enjoyment—and if you get the kids in on the action, you'll find that they are way more enthusiastic about eating something they help to prepare. And we're not talking hours and hours slaving away; the majority of Ayesha's recipes take only twenty to thirty minutes to make. You can find that time.

CREATE A ROUTINE. Good habits are just as easy to create as bad habits—and just as difficult to break! Once you've got a routine in place, the hard part is over. One way to do this is to create a checklist of the NEURO 9 foods you must eat every day: greens (such as spinach or arugula), whole grains (oatmeal or quinoa), seeds (flaxseeds), beans (black beans or chickpeas), berries (blueberries), nuts (walnuts or cashews), crucifers (broccoli or cauliflower), tea (green tea), herbs/spices (turmeric, cilantro, or mint). Then check off each food as you eat it, each day, and you'll have a daily routine that will help you eat the essential NEURO 9 foods every day—and track your success!

EATING HEALTHY AT WORK. Yes, Jen from Accounting isn't doing anybody any favors bringing in all those donuts. But you can't do anything about what *she* does—you can only help yourself. Start by taking food to work so that you're not relying on restaurants or cafeterias and so that you're already full of good, healthy food and those donuts don't look quite so appetizing. And do your best to eliminate stress at work (we know it isn't always possible) so that your amygdala doesn't go seeking sugar and fat—which won't help you get that project done any faster anyway. For that, you need your frontal lobe engaged, and it needs you to support it with healthy snacks.

EATING HEALTHY AT PARTIES. We're going to be real with you: for the next thirty days, don't go to any parties, or at least try not to. Once the thirty days are over, you don't have to say no to a piece of cake at your niece's birthday party. But you don't have to eat a giant slice, either. Take a small piece, eat a few bites, and then be done. This will be easier if you've had some healthy food first—which of course isn't always possible at parties. We have a kind of sneaky trick—we always eat a small, healthy meal before attending a party, and we always bring a healthy dish that we know everyone will enjoy.

RESTAURANTS. It's healthier to eat at home—you'll use less salt, you can be sure your food is organic, etc.—but sometimes it's nice to eat out, and there's no reason to deny yourself that pleasure. You can make smart, informed choices when you order, and make sure that at least half of your meal is greens and vegetables. You can also use our NEURO Plan Nutrition Spectrum (pages 68–69) to help you figure out the best option available.

THE NEURO PLAN NUTRITION SPECTRUM

This spectrum represents our extrapolation of the current research on nutrition and brain health. For us, it is not just about reflecting the science, but also speaking to the weight and context of the science. This food spectrum can serve as a useful tool, but is in no way perfectly representative of the complexity of nutrition science. So take it for what it is, a general guide open to change with new data or more complex interpretation.

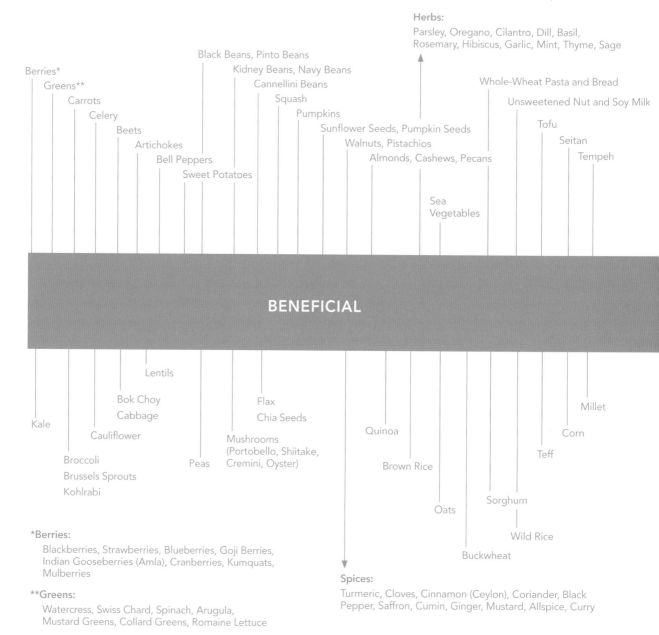

Herbs:
Parsley, Oregano, Cilantro, Dill, Basil, Rosemary, Hibiscus, Garlic, Mint, Thyme, Sage

Berries*
Greens**
Carrots
Celery
Beets
Artichokes
Bell Peppers
Sweet Potatoes

Black Beans, Pinto Beans
Kidney Beans, Navy Beans
Cannellini Beans
Squash
Pumpkins
Sunflower Seeds, Pumpkin Seeds
Walnuts, Pistachios
Almonds, Cashews, Pecans

Whole-Wheat Pasta and Bread
Unsweetened Nut and Soy Milk
Tofu
Seitan
Tempeh

Sea Vegetables

BENEFICIAL

Kale
Broccoli
Brussels Sprouts
Kohlrabi

Cauliflower

Bok Choy
Cabbage

Lentils

Peas

Mushrooms
(Portobello, Shiitake, Cremini, Oyster)

Flax
Chia Seeds

Quinoa

Brown Rice

Oats

Buckwheat

Sorghum

Wild Rice

Teff

Corn

Millet

*Berries:
Blackberries, Strawberries, Blueberries, Goji Berries, Indian Gooseberries (Amla), Cranberries, Kumquats, Mulberries

**Greens:
Watercress, Swiss Chard, Spinach, Arugula, Mustard Greens, Collard Greens, Romaine Lettuce

Spices:
Turmeric, Cloves, Cinnamon (Ceylon), Coriander, Black Pepper, Saffron, Cumin, Ginger, Mustard, Allspice, Curry

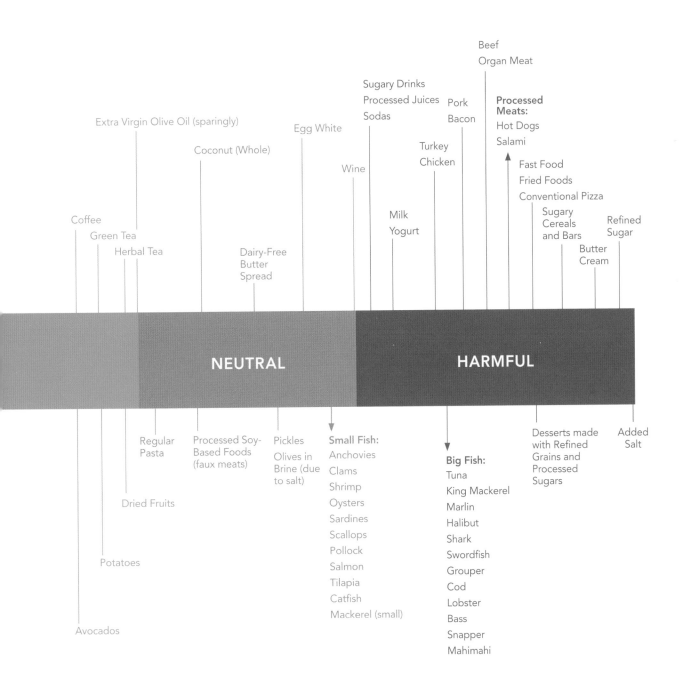

Beef
Organ Meat

Sugary Drinks
Processed Juices   Pork
Sodas   Bacon

Extra Virgin Olive Oil (sparingly)   Processed
                                              Meats:
                         Egg White   Hot Dogs
Coconut (Whole)   Salami

                                  Turkey   Fast Food
                          Wine   Chicken   Fried Foods
                                                        Conventional Pizza
Coffee   Sugary   Refined
                                    Milk   Cereals   Sugar
Green Tea   Yogurt   and Bars
                                                                 Butter
Herbal Tea   Dairy-Free   Cream
                    Butter
                    Spread

NEUTRAL   **HARMFUL**

                Regular   Processed Soy-   Pickles   **Small Fish:**
                Pasta   Based Foods   Anchovies   Desserts made   Added
                           (faux meats)   Olives in   Clams   with Refined   Salt
                                            Brine (due Shrimp   Grains and
        Dried Fruits   to salt)   Oysters   Processed
                                                        Sardines   Sugars
                                            Big Fish: Scallops
                                            Tuna   Pollock
                                            King Mackerel Salmon
        Potatoes   Marlin   Tilapia
                                            Halibut   Catfish
                                            Shark   Mackerel (small)
                                            Swordfish
                                            Grouper
                                            Cod
                                            Lobster
                                            Bass
Avocados   Snapper
                                            Mahimahi

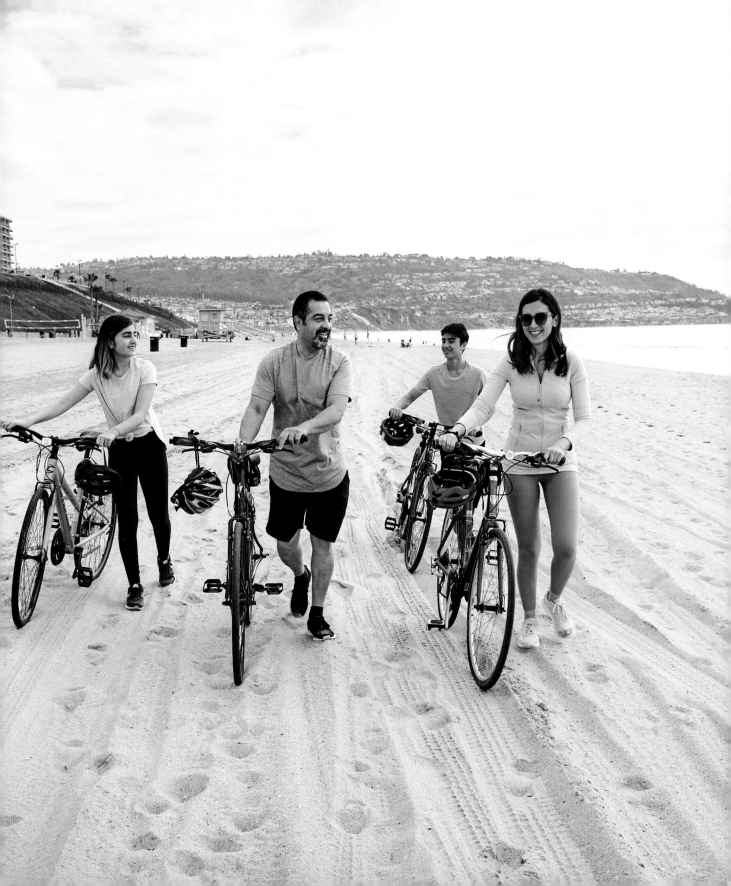

Part 3

THE NEURO PLAN: 30 DAYS OF BRAIN-BOOSTING

This is the beginning of a lifetime of brain vitality. And it only takes thirty days. It may seem a little intimidating, but we have some ideas for how to make it easier. We've put our heads together and come up with thirty days of the most optimal lifestyle changes for the most optimal brain. We have used SMART goals to ensure your success. Let's do this!

Now, if you have any underlying medical conditions, it's important to check with your doctor before undertaking the NEURO Plan. But this program is the beginning of living a brain-healthy lifestyle. Our goal is to help you get as close to total NEURO health as possible within these thirty days. These thirty days will be life-changing, and we're going to support you along the way, depending on your level of need.

Why thirty days? Because our research has taught us that thirty days is just about how long it takes to begin the process of first breaking and then creating habits. Doing something for just one week isn't enough, and two weeks isn't either. Committing fully for thirty days is the right amount of time to begin to alter your neural patterns, allowing you to form new habits.

> *With Alzheimer's or dementia, I trust exactly no one else ever.*
>
> —MICHAEL, AGE SEVENTY-THREE

WHAT'S IT GOING TO LOOK LIKE?

This isn't one of those plans where you have to follow strict daily instructions. For one thing, that just doesn't work—how are you going to create new habits if all you're doing is blindly following someone else's instructions? You're an adult—we don't need to hold your hand every day!

Another reason we aren't going to outline exact day-to-day meal plans or exercise plans is because we know everyone is coming to this plan from a different place. Some of you are already eating a plant-based diet, while others of you are going to need to avail yourselves of some of our swaps to replace your meat and cheese cravings. Some of you run marathons, while others work at a desk all day. Everybody has different starting points, resources, and tendencies, so we give you a set of guidelines that allows you to find where you are. These guidelines might be different from what you're used to, but they serve as an important framework toward your ultimate brain health. We guarantee that if you commit to truly finding yourself in the framework of the NEURO Plan for these thirty days, you will change your brain, and ultimately your life, for the better.

We offer you samples of what we believe an ideal week looks like under the NEURO Plan. This is the gold standard, folks—we're not holding anything back. These suggested weekly plans cover each aspect of NEURO—Nutrition, Exercise, Unwind, Restore, and Optimize—and each of them represents the ideal.

We laid out the rules in Part 1. We gave you the reasoning in Part 2. Now it's up to you to incorporate these rules into your daily life, in a way that works *for you.*

A WEEK OF THE NEURO LIFE: NUTRITION

All of the recipes we include in this book were created by Ayesha with optimal brain health in mind. Each of them includes one or more of the NEURO 9 and often some of our Thoughtful Twenty brain-nourishing foods, as well. You can definitely create your own recipes, but these are here to help make things a little easier over the course of the thirty days.

Day 1

BREAKFAST: Overnight Cinnamon Oats (page 106)

LUNCH: Farro Tempeh Bowl (page 144)

SNACK: Asian Cucumber Salad with Spicy Green Tea Tangerine Dressing (page 188)

DINNER: Spinach Farro Salad with Blackberry Dressing (page 191)

SWEET TREAT: Berries and almonds

Day 2

BREAKFAST: Mediterranean Scrumptious Scramble (page 111)

LUNCH: Totally Possible Burgers (page 128)

SNACK: Walnuts and dark chocolate

DINNER: South of the Border Salad (page 197)

SWEET TREAT: Fruit salad

Day 3

BREAKFAST: Berry Amaranth Smoothie Bowl (page 97)

LUNCH: Shiitake Chickpea Bulgur Bowl (page 120)

SNACK: Almonds and dried apricots

DINNER: Cauliflower Crust Pizza with Tofu Ricotta and Arugula Pesto (page 136)

SWEET TREAT: A cup of pomegranate seeds

Day 4

BREAKFAST: Avocado toast with seeds

LUNCH: Kale Caesar! (page 186)

SNACK: Omega Muffins (page 219)

DINNER: Creamy Mushroom and Radicchio Pasta Bake (page 132)

SWEET TREAT: Berries and dark chocolate

Day 5

BREAKFAST: Mighty Smoothie Bowl (page 112)

LUNCH: Sushi Tempeh Bowl with Tamari-Ginger Dressing (page 151)

SNACK: Celery spread with peanut butter

DINNER: Superfood Pasta with Hummus Walnut Dressing (page 152)

SWEET TREAT: Berries and nuts

Day 6

BREAKFAST: Chickpea Omelet (page 99)

LUNCH: Pinto Bean Quesadilla with Chipotle Cashew Queso (page 126)

SNACK: Apples with almond butter

DINNER: Lentil and Roasted Butternut Squash Salad (page 202)

SWEET TREAT: Berries and banana slices

Cooking Tips

Storing your broccoli already chopped *increases* its nutritional value.

You can wash your greens and then store them in your salad spinner, in the fridge, ready to go.

Day 7

BREAKFAST: Golden Waffles with Strawberry Sauce (page 94)

LUNCH: Mexican Quinoa Chipotle Salad (page 189)

SNACK: Fruit

DINNER: Whole-Wheat Pasta with Plantastic Neuroplastic Meatballs (page 156)

SWEET TREAT: Dark Chocolate Orange Pistachio Truffles (page 223)

A WEEK OF THE NEURO LIFE: EXERCISE

Exercise will look different for everyone. Our goal is not to make all of you into weight lifters or marathon runners; our goal is to get you fit and *healthy*. But "fit" means different things for different people, particularly if you're just getting started on the road to optimal health.

Before starting any exercise program, talk to your health-care professional to address any possible health concerns. We provide options here—but many of you may not be used to exercising every day, or you may not feel like you have the time. We understand this. This suggested week is the ideal; it's what you should shoot for.

Day 1

Twenty to thirty minutes of cardio, until you're tired. This can include jogging, swimming, brisk walking—whatever gets your heart pumping. Whatever level of exercise you're used to doing, you should work your heart for twenty to thirty minutes—you want to be out of breath to the point that you have difficulty finishing a sentence.

Day 2

Twenty to thirty minutes of strength training, until you're tired. This can include weight lifting, squats, push-ups, etc. For some people this might mean thirty mini-squats; for others it might mean five push-ups and five squats. Again, the goal is to work your muscles to the point where you are tired.

Day 3

Twenty to thirty minutes of flexibility work. This can include yoga, stretching, dance—whatever keeps you limber so you don't get hurt. If you can do the splits, well, more power to you! If you're working to touch your toes, that's great, too. Make sure you increase your stretching work slowly, and don't hurt yourself.

Day 4

Twenty to thirty minutes of cardio, until you're tired.

Day 5

Twenty to thirty minutes of strength training, until you're tired. A low amount of weight with a high number of repetitions is better than a lot of weight with very few reps.

Day 6

Twenty to thirty minutes of flexibility work.

Day 7

Rest. Give your body a break. But that doesn't mean lying on your back all day. You should continue to walk and move throughout the day, just not strenuously.

A WEEK OF THE NEURO LIFE: UNWIND

Remember, there are two kinds of stress, and one of them is good! Good stress is what you might be experiencing right now, reading this book. It's what makes you try for that promotion, and makes you push yourself to be better. Bad stress, on the other hand, is stress that has been imposed on you, does not have an end to it, prevents you from doing the things you want or need to do, and makes you unwell. We all experience both kinds of stress, and we all need to get in the habit of counteracting bad stress to make room for good stress.

Day 1

Identify your stresses. Clearly label the ones that are bad—such as worrying about something you've been putting off doing or thinking about something you said to someone that you now regret. At the same time, think about what is or could be a good stress—any action that is complex and challenging for your mind. Your goal is to increase the good stress and reduce the bad.

Day 2

Do fifteen minutes of meditation, breathing mindfully, or taking a relaxing, focused walk. These kinds of actions are tools to help you calm

the mind, and they take some practice. We have found that doing these for fifteen minutes is ideal, because it's long enough to get some good practice in but not too long that it's hard to stick with it. That said, any amount of time that helps you quiet your mind is perfect.

Day 3

Write in a journal for twenty to thirty minutes, focusing on anything that has been causing bad stress. When bad stress is weighing on you, it's a good idea to take the time to write it out—literally. The act of examining the roots of your bad stress can go a long way toward finding strategies to relieve it—by addressing it directly, delegating it, postponing it, or getting rid of it altogether.

Day 4

Do fifteen minutes of meditation, breathing mindfully, or taking a relaxing, focused walk.

Day 5

Listen to relaxing music for twenty to thirty minutes—something that calms your mind but at the same time allows you to focus on the elements of what you're listening to.

Day 6

Write in a journal for twenty to thirty minutes.

Day 7

Do fifteen minutes of meditation, breathing mindfully, or taking a relaxing, focused walk.

A WEEK OF THE NEURO LIFE: RESTORE

Everything you do will be wasted if you don't get a good night's sleep. Sleep helps your body process and reap the benefits of all of the above, and a lack of sleep is hard on your brain. Here are seven best practices to help you achieve true, restful sleep.

One

Go to bed at the same time every night, and then get out of bed seven to eight hours later, at the same time every morning. Even if you're not sleeping for those full seven to eight hours at the beginning, you are conditioning your brain to know when it's supposed to go to sleep, helping to establish a healthy circadian rhythm.

Two

Put your phone, tablet, or laptop away and turn off the TV at least half an hour before going to bed. This will augment stage one of your sleep cycle (see Part 1), letting your brain know it's time to rest. Looking at a screen or blue light disrupts your circadian rhythms, and stimulating your brain right before trying to put it to rest is obviously not a great idea.

Three

Don't eat or drink anything for at least three hours before going to bed, and definitely don't eat high-energy foods, as they will keep you awake. If you must eat something, try a banana or a small bowl of oatmeal, which won't rev up your systems. Your body's digestive processes need to be well underway before attempting to sleep; don't give your body a boost of energy before bed. And please, don't drink coffee or other caffeinated drinks after 2 p.m.

Four

Read or listen to something soothing right before bed. Unlike device screens, books have a natural soporific effect. That said, murder mysteries or thrillers probably aren't all that conducive to restful sleep, so maybe save those for another time.

Five

Check your room for too much light, noise, or other distractions. Do you have pets that disturb your sleep? Maybe they shouldn't be in your room at night. Do you need blinds to keep the streetlight out? Do you need some white noise in the background to drown out the noise in the neighborhood? Pay attention to what might be keeping you awake, and set yourself up for a good night's sleep.

Six

Wake up early to take a brisk walk just as the sun is coming up. Nothing is better for those circadian rhythms than this. Getting your body moving just as the sun is starting to rise is the best way to align your body's clock with that of the earth.

Seven

If you have trouble falling asleep, don't take naps during the day. Taking naps, especially after 3 p.m., throws your circadian rhythm off and resets your sleep cycle in a way that your brain has a hard time turning "off" when it's bedtime. So even if you are very tired during the day, don't nap. Your brain will adjust in a few days, and you will fall into a regimented sleep cycle.

Cooking Tips

You don't lose nutritional value when eating frozen vegetables or fruits. As a matter of fact, they may be *more* nutritious, as they are picked when ripe and then flash-frozen. You can keep them on hand at all times, without worrying that they'll spoil.

When you go grocery shopping, stock up on the ingredients you need for each recipe for the entire week. Make a shopping list and stick to it. This kind of planning will help you avoid those impulse purchases—which usually tend to be processed foods and sweets.

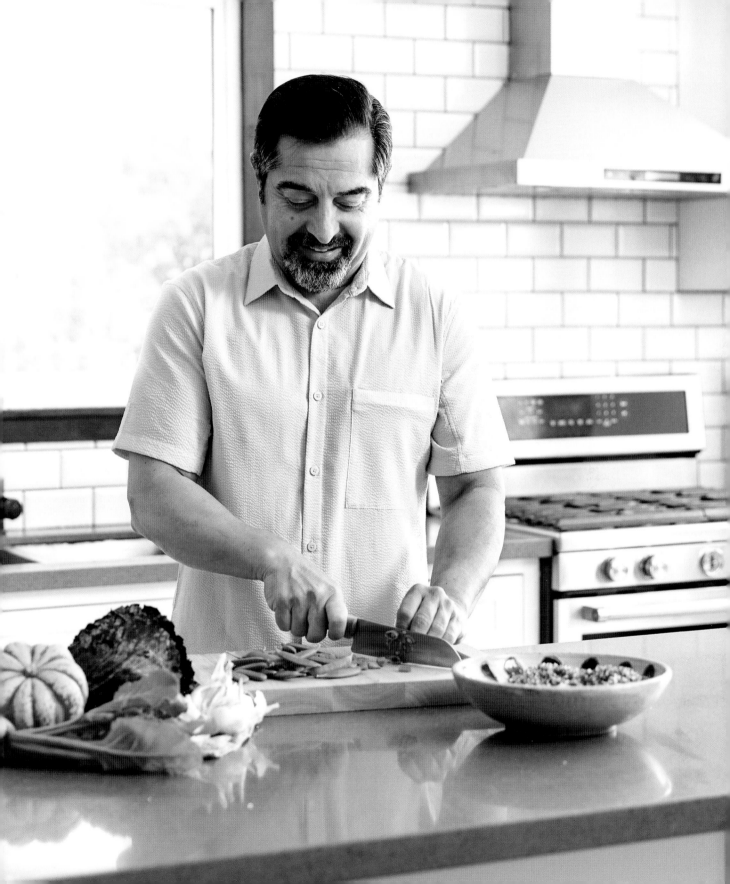

A WEEK OF THE NEURO LIFE: OPTIMIZE

Boost your cognitive reserve and increase your neuronal connections! Your brain works better when you stimulate it by doing cognitively challenging things that you enjoy.

Day 1

Spend at least an hour doing something engaging that you enjoy—paint, knit, sew, play chess, dance, or play an instrument. You want to do something challenging, but "enjoy" is important: if you dislike doing something, it's no longer a good stress—instead it becomes a bad stress, which we definitely don't want.

Day 2

Institute a no-phones rule during mealtimes. Putting your phone away will allow conversation and engage both the mind and the body. Pick a topic that encourages thought and a lively discussion. If you're on your own, listen to a podcast of something that excites or interests you (perhaps our podcast, *Brain Health and Beyond*), and something that makes you think.

Day 3

Call a friend you haven't talked to in a long time. Relationships are important, but they can be hard to hold on to with so many distractions in our lives. Take the time to focus on someone you care about—your brain and your heart will thank you.

Day 4

Like Day 1, spend at least an hour doing something engaging that you enjoy.

Day 5

Invite friends or family over for dinner and conversation. The best way to eat well is to do it with people you love, but be prepared to talk about a movie you all saw or a book you may all have read. A structured conversation forces you to go deep and draw on specifics and ideas, as opposed to generalities.

Day 6

Take a class or workshop that interests you—learn to paint or play an instrument, or learn a new language. Remember, challenge yourself, but also make sure you enjoy this.

Day 7

Like Day 1, spend at least an hour doing something engaging that you enjoy.

SO HOW AM I GOING TO FEEL?

Everyone will feel differently as they move through the thirty days of the NEURO Plan. But here are some common things that you might expect. Rest assured that you aren't the only one feeling a particular way.

DAY 1. I feel excited, prepared . . . maybe a little anxious that I might settle back into my previous habits, that it's going to be difficult because it's complex and comprehensive, not just adding or removing something in my life. I'm worried that I might not like the food, that my choices are limited, that I might not gain much with my brain health—but overall I know I've got this!

WEEK 1. I'm feeling a little low-energy, with slight headaches, and I'm always hungry. Also, I don't really like the taste of this food, and sometimes my stomach feels upset.

WEEK 2. My energy is starting to come back up, my digestive system has calmed down, and I'm not feeling hungry all the time. I'm still not completely on board with the change of food, and I'm really craving sugar.

WEEK 3. I feel pretty good. My body just *feels better*. I feel lighter, I have more energy, I don't feel tired as much, and I'm sleeping better. I feel more focused and alert. The cravings are still there, but I'm making new, easy meals that fill me up. I'm starting to look forward to foods that help me feel this way.

WEEK 4. My energy levels remain high, and I have more interest in doing interesting things—my mind doesn't turn immediately to social media or sinking into the couch to watch TV or whatever the easiest thing is. I'm not as forgetful as I was, and I can recall things better than I could a few weeks ago. I'm hungry for a challenge and not so hungry for sweets or meats anymore. Food tastes better, and I'm surprised how many fruits and vegetables I'm eating!

DAY 30. I did it! I feel *amazing*. My focus and attention have improved drastically! My memory has definitely improved and people around me have noticed. I'm less anxious and feel more relaxed and in control. I know that I can do this, and I understand the difference it's going to make in my brain and in my life.

GETTING READY

It takes a little bit of preparation to get started, and the first thing is some housekeeping.

Clean Out Your Refrigerator and Pantry

Your refrigerator and pantry are the source of all the food in your home, so you want to make sure they're set up to support you. Now, if you're anything like us, you may have plenty of good food in there, but you can't find it or you forget it's there! Nothing is more frustrating than wanting a healthy snack and grabbing a less-than-healthy one instead because you can't quickly find anything better. And haven't we all thrown out delicious produce we spent our hard-earned money on and then left to rot, forgotten, in a corner of the fridge?

Regular reorganization can help with that. Start by throwing out anything you can no longer use, either because it's past its expiration date or because it no longer aligns with your eating habits. Take the time to chop up your vegetables, placing them in clear glass containers so you can see what you've got. This helps you find things, makes it easier to start cooking, *and* makes sure you've got a handy healthy snack ready when you want it. Keep your various types of foods together in groups:

- Condiments or garnish, like kimchi, sauerkraut, hummus, nut butters, homemade salad dressings, sauces, and fruit-only jams (see recipe for Chia Berry Jam, page 210)
- Soy, cashew, or any plant milk
- Vegetables, chopped
- Vegetables, unchopped
- Fruits
- Berries
- Salad mix
- Herbs
- Lemons, limes, ginger, and garlic
- Breads
- Nut cheeses

> ### Cooking Tip
>
> Buy single-serving packets of already-cooked frozen brown rice, quinoa, cauliflower rice, and more for those days when you just can't handle the effort of turning on the stove.

If anything, our freezers are often *worse* than our refrigerators in terms of organization. Go through and throw out things you've forgotten about, and then organize so this doesn't happen again (for a while, anyway!), again, organizing by group:

- Frozen vegetables
- Frozen fruits
- Veggie burgers
- Cooked whole grains
- Herbs and spices

Go Shopping

There's good news here. Unlike some other diet and health programs, we're not expecting you to go out and buy a ton of expensive and weird products. We've got a family to feed, too, and like everybody else we work on a budget.

We also don't expect you to buy all thirty days' worth of food right up front. But there are some things that it's a good idea to have on hand before you start, since you're likely to need them fairly often:

- Canned no salt added beans, including chickpeas and black beans
- A variety of nuts, like walnuts and cashews

- A variety of spices, like cumin, cinnamon, paprika, chili powder
- Oats
- Quinoa
- Flaxseeds and chia seeds
- Brown rice

Make Time

All the parts of NEURO are going to take some time. You're going to be cooking, exercising, sleeping, and spending time with friends, so you need to clear some space in your calendar. But you'll find that it's a lot easier than you think. If you cut out TV time in the evenings, or time you spend on your phone or the internet, or time you spend lying awake feeling stressed about work—and we can relate!—you'll be surprised to discover how much time you have to spare.

But it does require some planning. If you're going to cook dinner, you'll want to make sure you have enough time to do that, that the shopping and some of the preparation is already done. If you're going to exercise, maybe you need to get up a little earlier in the morning—which might mean going to bed earlier, too. These are just some of the ways you'll adjust as you create new habits.

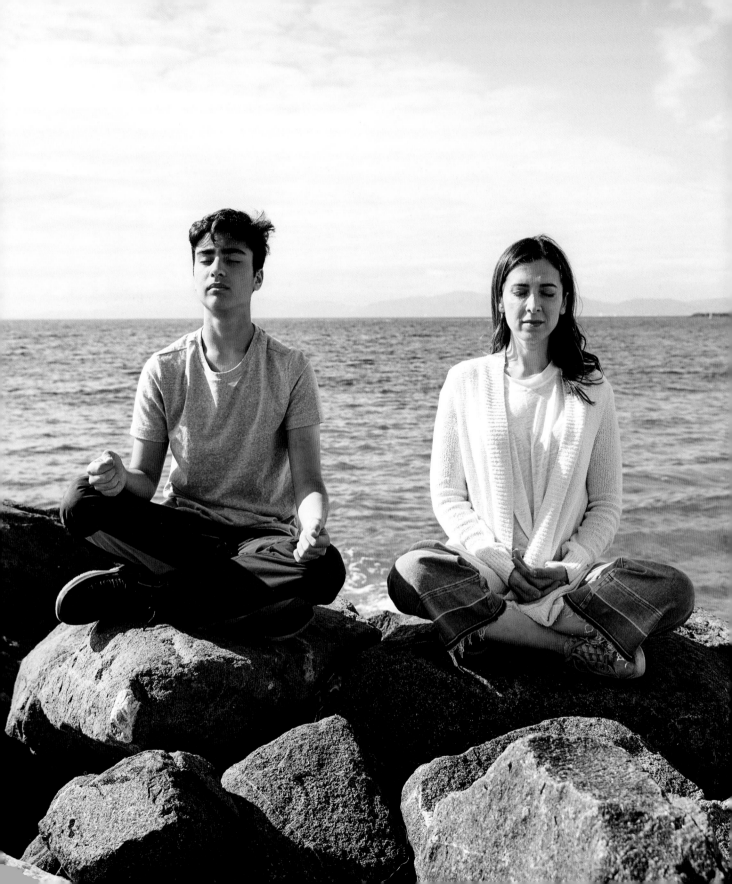

THIRTY DAYS LATER: YOU DID IT!

We wanted to present the thirty-day all-or-nothing NEURO Plan in order to make it simple for you. We wanted you to experience life in this black-and-white, rules-based way for thirty days so you could really give it your best shot. But we've got some great news for you: health isn't a black-and-white kind of thing, and neither is doing the work of *improving* your health.

Because here's the thing. Every tiny increment of positive change makes an enormous difference to your brain. We worked on a study that looked at 133,000 people over a period of twenty-five years.[14] We looked at their diets going back over time, and a great number of them had different degrees of a plant-centered diet, varying from minimal plants to 100 percent fully plant-based. Their successes were stratified to match their varying diets, and what we didn't expect was that each tiny step resulted in significantly better brain health.

Imagine walking down a road: one step after another gets you there, and no step gets you farther than any other, right? But for the journey toward health, this isn't so! One step takes you one step forward. But the second step takes you four steps forward, and the third step takes you nine steps forward, and so on, because the positive effects of even the smallest changes have an enormous impact. The cumulative effects of changing each of the aspects of NEURO when doing them *together* are so much greater than changing any one of them by themselves—so the added benefits of Nutrition, Exercise, Unwind, Restore, and Optimize are so much greater than each of them alone.

This was very encouraging and is in accord with what we have consistently seen in our careers—anyone, at any point in his or her journey toward cognitive health, can see profound improvement.

Now, this doesn't mean we're telling you that it's fine to go back to doing things like "eating in moderation" or to throw out our entire NEURO program! The way of life we've outlined for you, and that you've practiced over thirty days, is the ultimate goal.

But we do recognize that it may take some time to get there—and that is completely fine.

If you didn't do everything perfectly over these thirty days, don't worry too much about it. The last thing we want is for you to beat yourselves up and think that just because you couldn't do this immediately, you aren't capable of change. You are capable of change.

To set up some foundations for yourself to create lasting change—and to really work toward sustaining the ideal that was represented by these thirty days—let's look again at SMART goals (see Part 2).

SMART GOALS

SMART goals will get you there, one step at a time. These thirty days were like asking a baby to try to run before she's learned to crawl. SMART goals will help you meet yourself where you are, wherever you are.

S = SPECIFIC. Choose a specific action. What are you going to address? Don't say "I'm going to eat a perfect diet," because that's way too broad. Instead, try something like "I'm going to eat more greens."

M = MEASURABLE. But then, refine that goal. What does "more" mean? More could be one leaf of lettuce, if you never, ever eat salad, and that won't do you much good. Change your goal from "I'm going to eat more greens" to "I'm going to eat five servings of greens per week."

A = ATTAINABLE. Can you really do that? Don't set yourself a goal that you know you won't attain. What would be the point? The whole idea here is to give you a burst of endorphins of joy in your own achievement. Can you eat five servings of greens in a week? *Will* you?

R = RELEVANT. Double-check that goal. Is it aligned with your desire for better cognitive health?

T = TIME BOUND. Make sure your goal has an end date—because how else will you know that you've succeeded? Make the goal "I'm going to eat five servings of greens every week for four weeks." That way, when those four weeks are up, you'll be able to bask in your success.

REWARDS

Whatever you do, make sure to take the time to reward yourself. You've finished the thirty days of the NEURO Plan; how are you going to celebrate?

Think carefully about this, and be intentional about it. For instance, as we said before, it's probably not a great idea to reward yourself by having a "cheat day" or eating a donut. This just keeps you in a mindset of deprivation, a way of thinking that you can get to the "good" food only by walking over the hot coals of eating "health food."

But this isn't the case. The more you eat a brain-healthy, plant-based diet, the more you will come to genuinely enjoy and crave such foods—but not if you periodically slather your taste buds with oversugared, oversalted, over-processed "fake food."

So instead of rewarding yourself with food—which will only make it harder for you to succeed at your SMART goals—reward yourself with something that will help you continue on your journey toward cognitive health. For completing your first thirty days, maybe have a dinner party to celebrate this huge success, inviting friends and family to share a delicious, healthy meal. Maybe go out dancing. Maybe take a day trip somewhere.

But make sure you celebrate smaller successes, too, such as achieving a SMART goal. Every success is worth celebrating, because every success has an enormous impact on your health.

We are so proud of you. We know this isn't easy—we've been through it ourselves! It takes hard work, and it takes the support of a community. We are here to help you and wish you all the best of NEURO health.

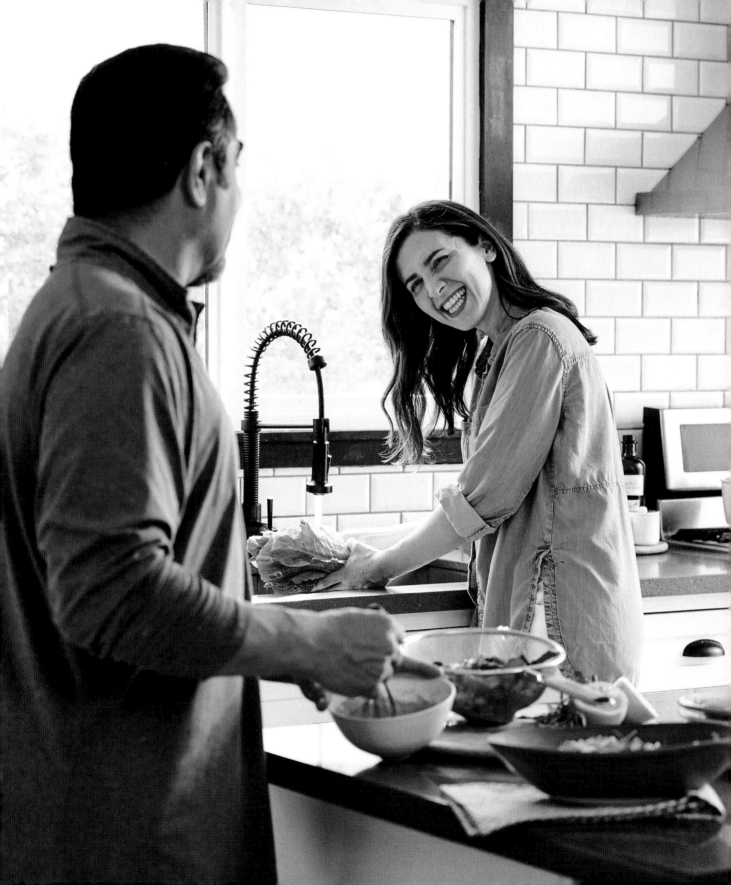

RECIPES

Vitalizing **VEGGIES AND** *Brain-Gain* **GRAINS**

Synaptic **SOUPS AND SALADS**

Dreamy DIPS AND DRESSINGS

Neuroprotective NUT CHEESES

Mindful MUFFINS AND *Stimulating* SCONES

Dopamine-Boosting DESSERTS

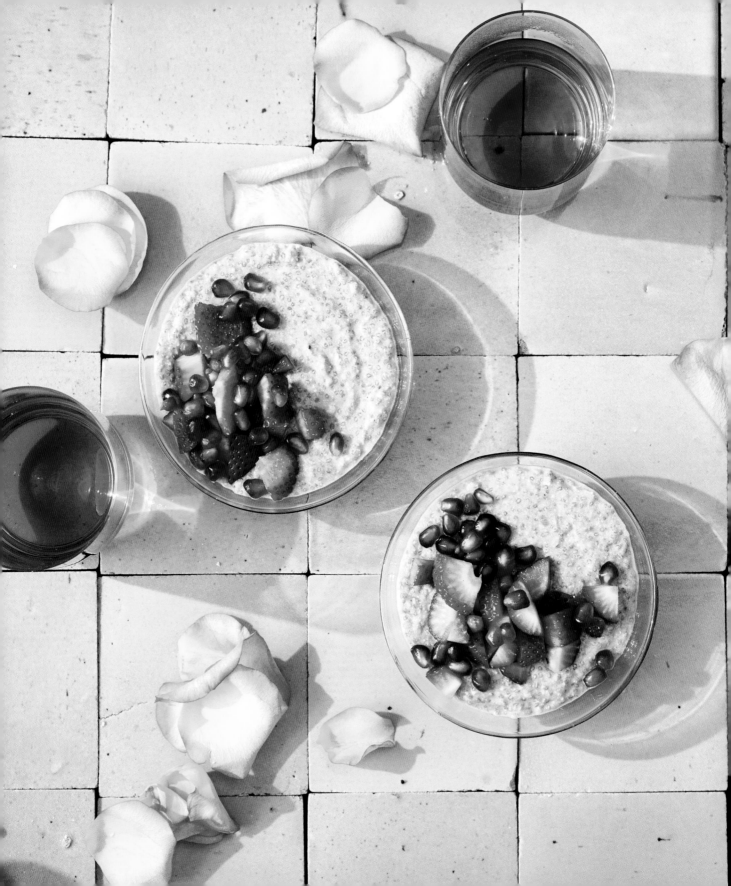

STRAWBERRY ROSE CHIA PUDDING

⅔ cup hulled and chopped fresh strawberries or chopped frozen strawberries

1 tablespoon lemon juice

1 teaspoon rosewater (or to taste)

1½ cups unsweetened cashew milk or other plant milk of choice

3 tablespoons monk fruit sweetener (or to taste)

⅓ cup raw cashews, soaked in boiling water for at least 30 minutes or in room-temperature water overnight

¼ cup chia seeds (white chia seeds, if possible)

OPTIONAL GARNISHES

⅓ cup chopped fresh strawberries

2 tablespoons pomegranate seeds or goji berries or 2 tablespoons unsalted toasted cashews, chopped

NEURO 9 ITEMS: strawberries, cashews, chia seeds

PREP TIME: 10 minutes, not including the 30 minutes of soaking

COOKING TIME: none

TOTAL TIME: 10 minutes plus time to chill

YIELD: 3 servings

In a blender, blend strawberries, lemon juice, rosewater, cashew milk, monk fruit sweetener, and cashews until smooth.

Stir in chia seeds and divide among three small glasses or jars. Refrigerate until set (about 2 hours), stirring after about 15 minutes to distribute the chia seeds evenly.

If desired, serve the puddings topped with fresh strawberries and pomegranate seeds, or toasted cashews.

Refrigerate tightly covered for up to two days.

GOLDEN WAFFLES WITH STRAWBERRY SAUCE

NEURO 9 ITEMS: strawberries, cashews, chia seeds

PREP TIME: 10 minutes

COOKING TIME: 15 minutes

TOTAL TIME: 25 minutes

YIELD: 3 waffles

FOR THE STRAWBERRY SAUCE

1 cup strawberries, sliced

Juice and zest of 1 small lemon

2 tablespoons monk fruit sweetener (optional)

2 to 3 tablespoons water

FOR THE WAFFLES

2 tablespoons flaxseeds

3 tablespoons water

1 cup 100% whole-wheat flour

⅔ cup oat flour

1½ teaspoons baking powder

½ teaspoon ground turmeric

2 tablespoons arrowroot flour

¼ teaspoon salt

⅓ cup unsweetened applesauce

1 teaspoon apple cider vinegar

1¼ cups unsweetened soy milk (as needed)

Avocado oil spray

Add strawberries, lemon juice, lemon zest, sweetener (if desired), and water to a small saucepan and bring to a boil over medium heat. Cover partially, reduce the heat, and let simmer for about 10 to 12 minutes, or until the strawberries are very tender. Stir the mixture occasionally and add a splash of water if it becomes too thick. If you wish, purée using an immersion blender. Set aside.

Meanwhile, preheat a waffle iron to medium-high.

Mix flaxseeds with water in a small bowl and set aside.

Combine the whole-wheat flour, oat flour, baking powder, turmeric, arrowroot flour, and salt in a large bowl. Gently stir in the applesauce, apple cider vinegar, flaxseed mixture, and enough soy milk to get a thick batter. Do not overmix.

Spray the waffle iron with avocado oil cooking spray and pour about ½ cup batter in the center and cook until golden brown, following the manufacturer's instructions. Keep warm while you make the remaining waffles.

Serve with the strawberry sauce and any other desired toppings.

Recipe Notes

- *Freeze the waffles for up to one month.*

- *Top with some Coco-Hazelnut Butter (page 226).*

- *Refrigerate any leftover strawberry sauce in a sealed container for up to one week.*

- *Serve with fresh fruit, nut butters, or cashew cream, or with your choice of savory toppings.*

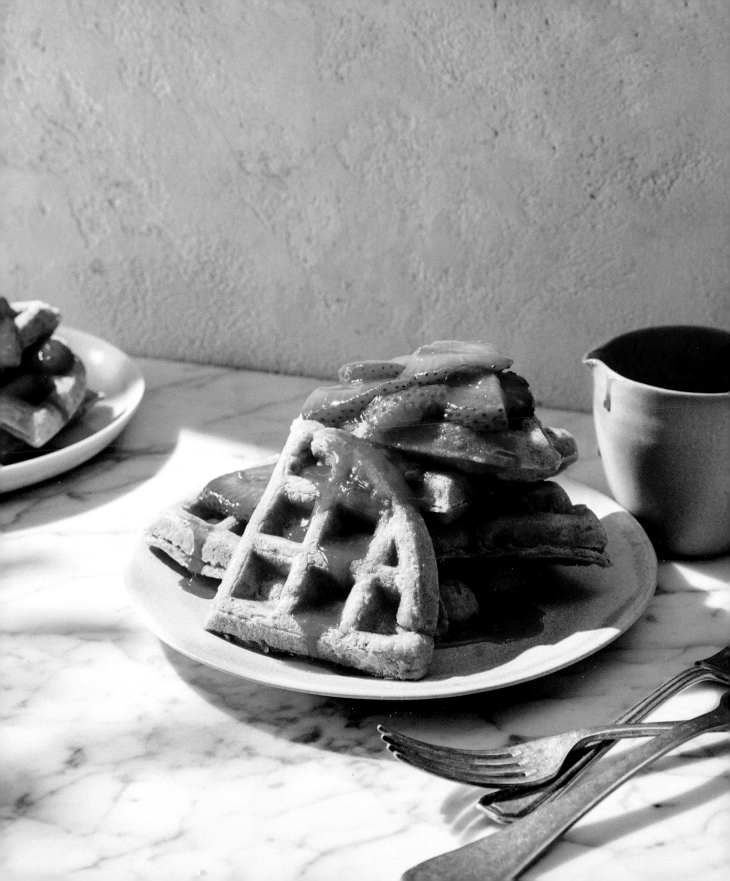

SWEET POTATO OAT PANCAKES

NEURO 9 ITEMS: oat flour, flaxseeds, spices

PREP TIME: 15 minutes

COOKING TIME: 15 minutes

TOTAL TIME: 30 minutes

YIELD: 6 pancakes

2 tablespoons ground flaxseeds

¼ cup water

¼ cup unsweetened applesauce

1 medium sweet potato or yam, boiled and mashed

1 cup oat milk or soy milk (as needed)

1 cup oat flour

3 teaspoons baking powder

⅓ cup tapioca starch

½ teaspoon each of ginger and cinnamon

2 tablespoons monk fruit sweetener (optional)

EVOO spray (optional)

OPTIONAL TO SERVE
Maple-flavored sugar-free monk fruit syrup and chopped pecans

Mix flaxseeds and water in a small bowl and set aside.

Blend applesauce, sweet potato, oat milk, and flaxseed mixture in a blender or food processor until smooth.

Combine oat flour, baking powder, tapioca starch, ginger, cinnamon, and sweetener in a large bowl and gently stir in the wet ingredients to get a smooth pancake batter (do not overmix). If necessary, adjust the consistency with a little milk or flour. Set aside for 5 minutes.

Heat a griddle or nonstick (or heavy-bottomed) skillet over medium heat and lightly spray with EVOO spray (optional, to make the surface nonstick). Working in batches, ladle the batter onto the griddle or skillet to form three pancakes, spacing them apart; cook for about 4 to 5 minutes, then flip over and cook for 3 to 4 minutes or until bubbly and golden. Transfer to a plate and keep warm. Repeat with the remaining batter. Serve immediately.

Recipe Notes

- *If desired, drizzle with maple-flavored sugar-free monk fruit syrup and sprinkle with chopped pecans.*

- *You can also serve with slices of banana or diced green apples.*

- *Serve with Chia Berry Jam (page 210).*

BERRY AMARANTH SMOOTHIE BOWL

NEURO 9 ITEMS: amaranth, berries, chia seeds

PREP TIME: 5 minutes

COOKING TIME: 20 minutes

TOTAL TIME: 25 minutes

YIELD: 3 servings

FOR THE SMOOTHIE

½ cup plus 1 tablespoon amaranth

1½ cups frozen mixed berries

1½ cups water

2 tablespoons chia seeds

2 tablespoons cacao powder

2 cups unsweetened plant-based milk, such as hemp, oat, or soy milk

Zest of 1 orange

FOR SERVING

3 tablespoons sunflower seeds

1 tablespoon puffed amaranth

⅓ cup strawberries, hulled and diced

Rinse the amaranth under cold running water and add to a small saucepan together with 1½ cups water; bring to a boil, reduce heat to low, and let simmer for 15 to 20 minutes or until the water has absorbed and the amaranth is tender. Set aside.

Add the cooked amaranth, berries, chia seeds, cacao powder, milk, and orange zest to a blender and blend until smooth (if too thick, adjust the consistency with more milk or water).

Divide the smoothie mixture among three bowls and garnish with sunflower seeds, puffed amaranth, and strawberries. Serve immediately.

Recipe Note

- *Lightly toast the amaranth for a fragrant, nutty flavor. Soaking it overnight will make it easier to digest and will bring out the nutrients.*

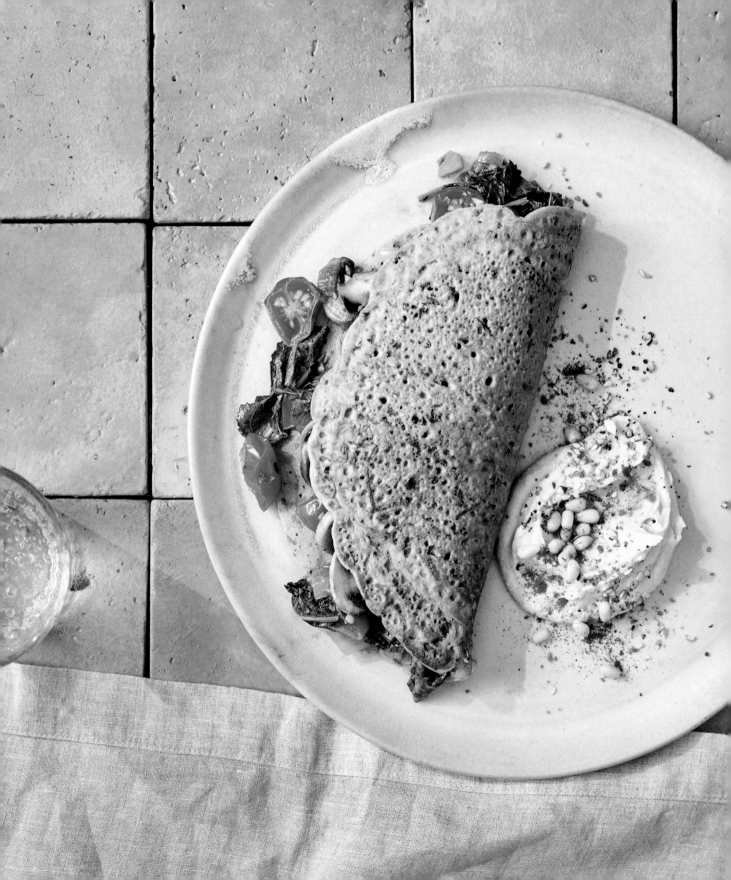

CHICKPEA OMELET

NEURO 9 ITEMS: chickpeas, herbs and spices

PREP TIME: 10 minutes

COOKING TIME: 10 minutes

TOTAL TIME: 20 minutes

YIELD: 3 servings

FOR THE CHICKPEA BATTER

1 cup chickpea/garbanzo bean flour

½ teaspoon baking powder

½ teaspoon paprika

½ teaspoon garlic powder

½ teaspoon turmeric powder

Salt and freshly ground black pepper, to taste

1 cup water plus 2 to 3 tablespoons to thin the batter if needed

1 teaspoon apple cider vinegar

¼ cup chopped chives

1 cup chopped parsley

VEGETABLES

EVOO spray

2 to 3 garlic cloves, chopped

½ red onion, finely chopped

2 cups cremini mushrooms, chopped

Salt and freshly ground black pepper, to taste

1 cup halved cherry tomatoes

2 cups spinach leaves

FOR THE BATTER: Place the dry ingredients in a large bowl. Mix well, then add water and apple cider vinegar, whisking them in. Add the chopped herbs to the batter. Mix well and set aside. The batter needs to resemble a pancake batter—thin enough to spread quickly.

FOR THE VEGETABLES: Heat a nonstick pan on medium-high. Spray with a little EVOO. Sauté the garlic for about 30 seconds. Then add the onion and sauté for 2 minutes. Add the mushrooms and stir for 2 minutes. Season with salt and pepper. Add the tomatoes and let everything cook together for about 3 minutes. Turn off the heat and add the spinach to wilt. Put all the cooked vegetables in a bowl and set aside. Clean your pan with a cloth or towel or rinse quickly.

FOR THE OMELET: Place the clean nonstick pan on medium-high heat. Once hot, spray with a little EVOO to make sure the batter does not stick to the pan (optional). Pour a third of the batter in the hot pan and spread into a round shape. Wait for 1 to 2 minutes and watch carefully for the edges to cook and small air bubbles to form on the top—that's when the omelet is ready to be flipped.

Flip the omelet using a large, broad spatula. Let it cook for another 1 to 2 minutes.

Place a third of the cooked vegetables on half of the omelet. Gently fold the other half on top of the vegetables. Make two more omelets. Serve immediately with hot sauce, hummus, or a side salad.

CRUSTLESS MINI QUICHES

NEURO 9 ITEMS: kale, chives, tahini, tofu, herbs and spices

PREP TIME: 10 minutes

COOKING TIME: 30 minutes

TOTAL TIME: 40 minutes

YIELD: 6 quiches

EVOO spray

¼ cup low-sodium vegetable broth or water (more as needed)

3 scallions, chopped

1 garlic clove, minced

1 medium red bell pepper, finely diced

1 cup trimmed and chopped asparagus

1 packed cup chopped baby kale or watercress

1 tablespoon each of chopped fresh chives and parsley

⅓ cup unsweetened plant-based milk, preferably soy (more as needed)

2 tablespoons tahini

1 8-ounce block silken tofu, drained

2½ tablespoons nutritional yeast

1½ tablespoons arrowroot flour (or 100% whole-wheat flour)

½ teaspoon turmeric

¼ teaspoon salt and freshly ground black pepper, to taste

Preheat the oven to 375°F. Spray a six-cup muffin pan with EVOO spray or line with paper muffin cups.

Heat a large skillet over medium-high heat and add 2 tablespoons broth, scallions, garlic, and bell pepper; cook until softened and fragrant, about 3 minutes. Stir in asparagus and cook for 2 minutes, adding 1 to 2 tablespoons broth as needed to prevent the mixture from sticking to the pan. Turn off the heat and mix in kale, chives, and parsley.

In a blender, blend together plant milk, tahini, tofu, nutritional yeast, arrowroot, and turmeric until smooth, and then stir into the vegetables. Season with salt and pepper to taste.

Divide the mixture among the prepared cups and bake for about 25 minutes, or until set and golden brown.

Cool the quiches in the pan for 5 to 10 minutes before serving.

Recipe Note

- *Experiment by adding different green or other vegetables in the batter.*

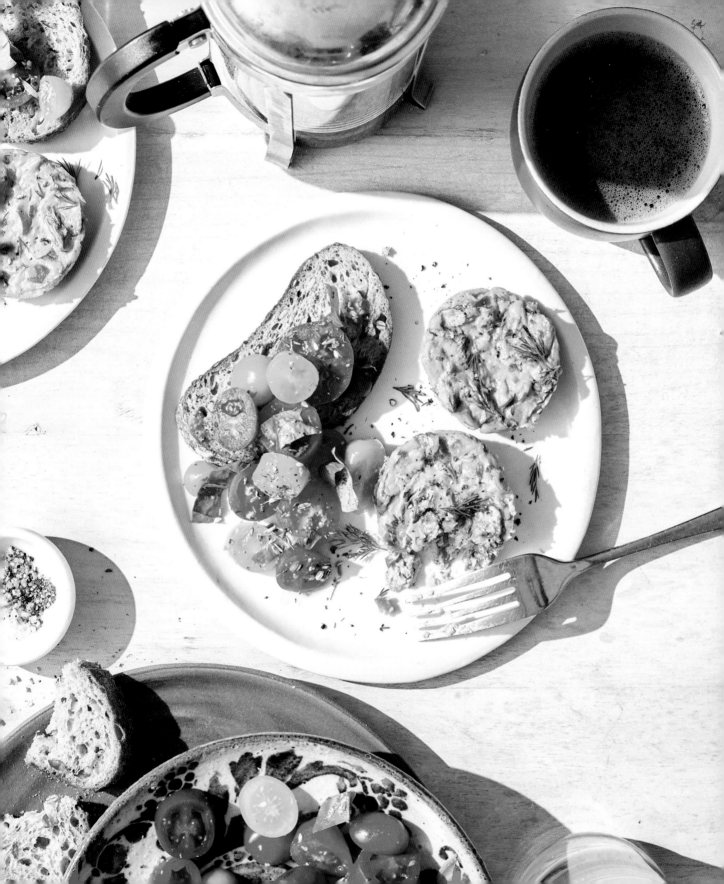

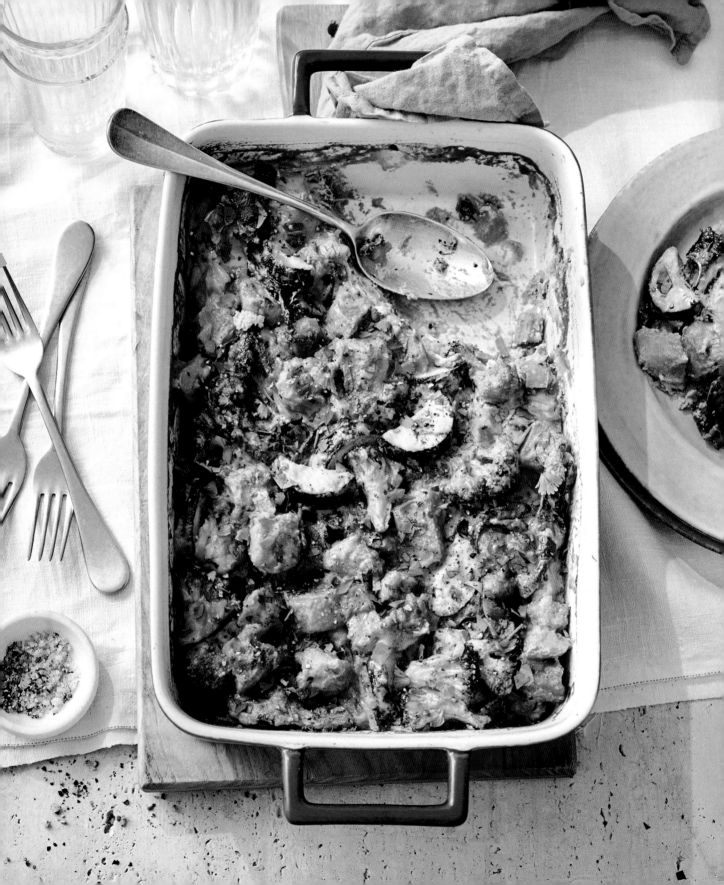

CHEESY TEMPEH AND SWEET POTATO BREAKFAST CASSEROLE

FOR THE CASHEW CHEESE SAUCE

1 cup raw cashews, soaked in boiling water for at least 30 minutes or in room-temperature water overnight

4 tablespoons nutritional yeast

1 teaspoon yellow miso paste

½ teaspoon garlic powder

½ teaspoon salt

1 cup hot water

FOR THE TEMPEH AND VEGETABLES

EVOO spray

⅓ cup low-sodium vegetable broth, divided

1 8-ounce package tempeh, cut into bite-size cubes or crumbled

2 tablespoons reduced-sodium tamari or liquid aminos

2 leeks, chopped

1 teaspoon finely grated ginger

2 garlic cloves, finely minced

1 medium sweet potato, cut into bite-size pieces

2 cups chopped broccoli florets

1 medium zucchini, cut into bite-size pieces

2 packed cups spinach

2 tablespoons finely chopped parsley or cilantro

Salt and freshly ground black pepper, to taste

NEURO 9 ITEMS: cashews, tempeh, broccoli, spinach

PREP TIME: 15 minutes, not including the 30 minutes of soaking

COOKING TIME: 45–50 minutes

TOTAL TIME: 60–65 minutes

YIELD: 6 servings

Preheat the oven to 350°F and lightly spray the bottom of a large casserole baking dish with EVOO spray.

Place all the cashew cheese sauce ingredients into a strong blender and process until velvety and smooth, adding more water if necessary to get a sauce consistency. Set aside.

Using a large nonstick pan, add 2 to 3 tablespoons broth and tempeh. Cover with lid and let tempeh steam for about 4 to 5 minutes. Remove cover and spray with EVOO. Continue cooking 5 minutes, stirring often, until lightly browned. Add tamari or liquid aminos and continue cooking for 1 to 2 minutes. Using a slotted spoon, transfer tempeh to a plate and set aside.

Add leeks, ginger, and garlic to the same pan and sauté for 2 to 3 minutes. Add the sweet potatoes and continue cooking for about 5 minutes, then add the broccoli. Cook, stirring occasionally, until just tender, adding a splash of broth to prevent sticking.

Stir in zucchini, spinach, parsley, and tempeh; season to taste, then tip the mixture into the prepared baking dish and spread evenly. Pour the cashew cheese sauce over all, mix gently, and smooth the top.

Bake for about 25 minutes, or until golden brown. Cool completely before cutting into squares and serving.

Recipe Note

- *You may prepare the casserole in advance and refrigerate until needed.*

BERRY WHOLE GRAIN SMOOTHIE BOWL

NEURO 9 ITEMS: quinoa, buckwheat, berries, kale, flaxseeds, cashew butter, spices

PREP TIME: 10 minutes

COOKING TIME: none

TOTAL TIME: 10 minutes

YIELD: 3 servings

⅓ cup cooked quinoa

⅓ cup cooked buckwheat

2 cups unsweetened cashew milk or other plant-based milk

2 cups fresh or frozen blackberries

1 ripe avocado, pitted and skinned

2 cups spinach or baby kale

1 teaspoon flaxseeds

2 tablespoons unsalted cashew butter or other nut butter

¼ teaspoon cardamom

Monk fruit sweetener to taste (optional)

A cup of ice cubes (optional)

FOR SERVING

⅓ cup fresh blackberries

3 tablespoons chopped cashews or other nuts of choice

Combine quinoa, buckwheat, and cashew milk in a blender and blend at high speed until smooth. Add blackberries, avocado, spinach, flaxseeds, cashew butter, cardamom, and monk fruit sweetener, if using. You may also add a handful of ice cubes. Blend until smooth. Adjust the consistency to taste with extra milk or water.

Divide the smoothie among three serving bowls and top with blackberries and chopped cashews. Serve immediately.

Recipe Note

- *Add crunch by topping the smoothie with some Memory-Boosting Granola (page 109).*

ZUCCHINI CHICKPEA SAVORY PANCAKES

NEURO 9 ITEMS: chickpea flour, herbs and spices

PREP TIME: 15 minutes

COOKING TIME: 20 minutes

TOTAL TIME: 35 minutes

YIELD: 6 pancakes

1¼ cups chickpea flour

¼ teaspoon each of ground cumin, turmeric, garlic powder, and paprika

1½ tablespoons nutritional yeast

½ teaspoon baking powder

¼ teaspoon salt

1 jalapeño, seeds and pith removed, finely chopped

2 tablespoons each of fresh cilantro and dill

3 scallions, finely chopped

1 small zucchini or summer squash, grated

1 to 1½ cups water (as needed)

Sea salt and freshly ground black pepper, to taste

EVOO spray for cooking

OPTIONAL GARNISHES

Salsa, sliced tomatoes, arugula, spring mix, sliced cucumbers, and hot sauce

Mix chickpea flour, spices, nutritional yeast, baking powder, and salt in a large mixing bowl. Combine jalapeño, cilantro, dill, scallions, and zucchini in another bowl and add to the dry mixture. Whisk in enough water to get a pancake-like batter. Season with salt and pepper and set aside.

Heat a nonstick skillet over medium heat and spray with EVOO. Use a measuring cup to scoop out ½ cup batter, pour onto the skillet, and using a spatula quickly spread to the desired thickness. Cook for about 1 to 2 minutes per side, or until nicely browned. Repeat with the remaining batter.

Serve warm with any of the toppings. Wrap any leftover pancakes and refrigerate for up to two days. Reheat before serving.

Recipe Note

- *Serve with Cashew Sour Cream (recipe on page 205), or Spicy Green Hummus (page 206).*

OVERNIGHT CINNAMON OATS

NEURO 9 ITEMS: oats, spices, flaxseeds, sunflower seeds, hemp seeds, walnuts, berries

PREP TIME: 5 minutes

COOKING TIME: none

TOTAL TIME: 5 minutes plus overnight soaking

YIELD: 3 servings

1½ cups old-fashioned oats

2 teaspoons ground cinnamon

1½ tablespoons flaxseeds

2 tablespoons sunflower seed butter (or any nut butter)

2 tablespoons hemp seeds

1 tablespoon monk fruit sweetener (optional)

1½ cups unsweetened plant-based milk, preferably soy (more as needed)

2 tablespoons sunflower seeds

2 tablespoons coarsely chopped pecans or walnuts

1 cup blueberries, sliced strawberries, or any fruit of choice

Combine oats, cinnamon, flaxseeds, sunflower seed butter, hemp seeds, and monk fruit sweetener, if using, in an airtight container (a mason jar works well). Slowly add the milk, stirring. Cover with a lid and refrigerate overnight.

When ready to serve, stir the oats and add more plant milk if needed. Top with the sunflower seeds, pecans, walnuts, and berries or other fruits.

Recipe Note

* *Explore different flavors by adding other spices such as nutmeg, cardamom, or a pinch of saffron. Add a tablespoon of cacao to the mixture before soaking for a chocolate flavor.*

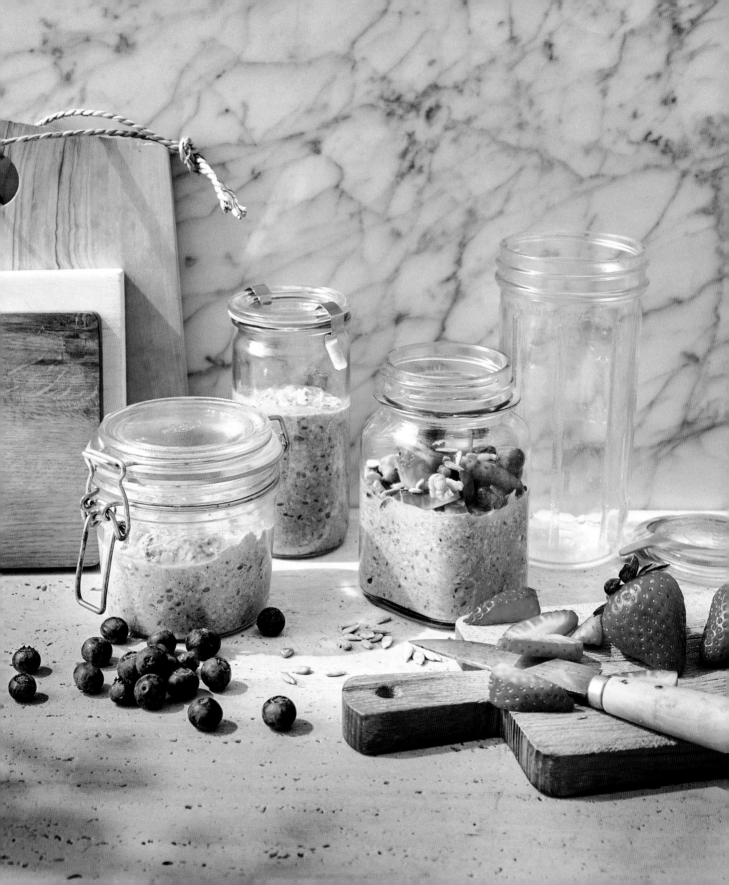

BAKED BERRY PANCAKES

NEURO 9 ITEMS: flaxseeds, 100% whole-wheat flour, almond butter, blueberries

PREP TIME: 5 minutes

COOKING TIME: 12 minutes

TOTAL TIME: 17 minutes

YIELD: 6 pancakes

1 tablespoon ground flaxseeds

3 tablespoons water

1 cup 100% whole-wheat flour

3 tablespoons arrowroot flour

1 to 2 tablespoons monk fruit sweetener (optional)

½ teaspoon baking powder

¼ teaspoon baking soda

⅛ teaspoon salt

1 tablespoon unsalted almond butter or other nut butter of choice

¾ cup unsweetened almond or other nondairy milk of choice (or as needed)

2 teaspoons apple cider vinegar or lemon juice

3 tablespoons fresh blueberries or dairy-free and sugar-free dark chocolate chips

Preheat the oven to 375°F and line a large baking sheet with parchment paper or a silicone baking mat.

Mix flaxseeds and water in a small bowl and set aside.

Combine all dry ingredients in a large mixing bowl and add flaxseed mixture, almond butter, almond milk, and apple cider vinegar; whisk until smooth, adding more milk if necessary to get a pancake batter consistency. Stir in the blueberries or chocolate chips.

Using a measuring spoon, scoop out 2½ heaped tablespoons batter and spread on the baking sheet to form a 3½- to 4-inch circle. Repeat for a total of six circles.

Bake, flipping halfway through, for about 12 minutes, or until the pancakes are golden.

Serve warm with toppings of choice.

Recipe Notes

- *Add flavor by adding ½ teaspoon cinnamon or 1 teaspoon lemon or orange zest to the batter.*

- *If you prefer, cook the pancakes in a skillet or on a griddle for about 4 minutes per side.*

MEMORY-BOOSTING GRANOLA

NEURO 9 ITEMS: oats, nuts, quinoa, pumpkin seeds, hemp seeds, chia seeds, tahini, spices

PREP TIME: 5 minutes

COOKING TIME: 35 minutes

TOTAL TIME: 40 minutes

YIELD: 10 servings (5 cups)

2 cups rolled oats

⅔ cup mixed raw nuts, such as macadamia nuts, cashews, walnuts, or pistachios, coarsely chopped

⅓ cup slivered raw almonds

⅔ cup quinoa flakes or uncooked white quinoa

¼ cup pumpkin seeds

¼ cup hemp seeds

¼ cup chia seeds

1 teaspoon ground cinnamon

½ teaspoon ground cardamom (optional)

⅓ cup tahini (or smooth sugar-free peanut butter)

2 teaspoons vanilla extract

Zest of 1 orange (optional)

Preheat the oven to 300°F; line two large, rimmed baking sheets with silicone baking mats or parchment paper and set aside.

Mix oats, mixed nuts, almonds, quinoa, pumpkin seeds, hemp seeds, chia seeds, cinnamon, and cardamom in a large bowl. Stir tahini, vanilla extract, and orange zest, if using, in a small bowl and drizzle over the dry mixture, stirring until combined.

Spread the mixture evenly onto the prepared baking sheets and bake, stirring halfway, until lightly toasted, about 35 minutes.

Let granola cool to room temperature before storing in an airtight container for up to two weeks.

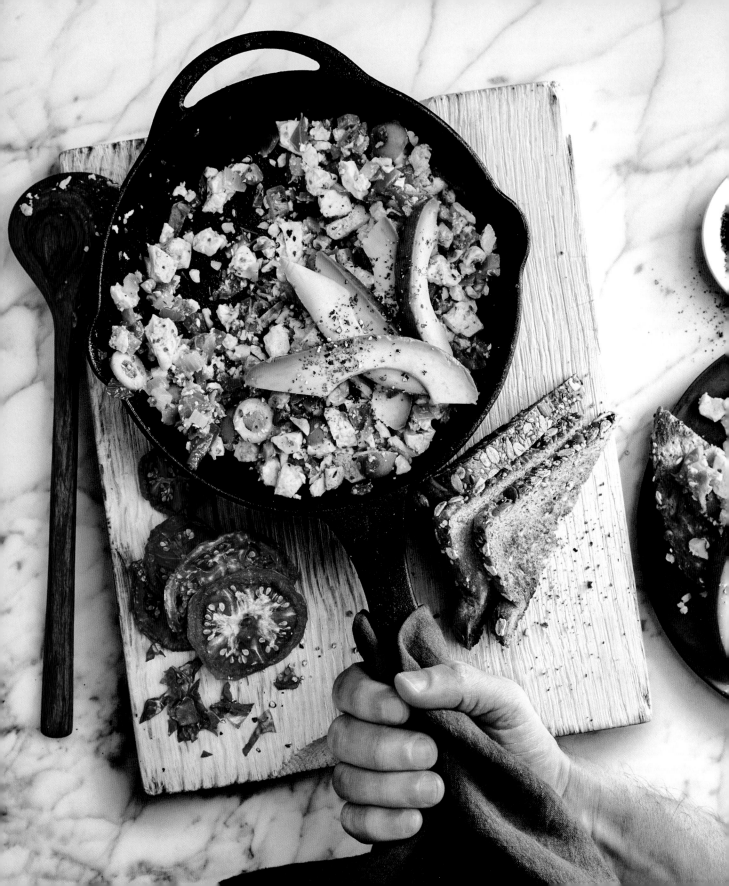

MEDITERRANEAN SCRUMPTIOUS SCRAMBLE

NEURO 9 ITEMS: tofu, walnuts, herbs and spices

PREP TIME: 10 minutes

COOKING TIME: 15 minutes

TOTAL TIME: 20 minutes

YIELD: 3 servings

1 tablespoon EVOO

2 tablespoons low-sodium vegetable broth (more as needed)

½ medium red onion, finely chopped

¼ cup sundried tomatoes soaked in water, chopped

¼ cup pitted sliced green olives

2 garlic cloves, crushed

1 14-ounce block extra-firm tofu, drained and crumbled into small bite-size pieces

1 teaspoon ground turmeric

1 tablespoon oregano

Sea salt and freshly ground black pepper, to taste

3 tablespoons nutritional yeast

Handful of fresh basil leaves, shredded

1 avocado, pitted and sliced

3 tablespoons walnuts, roughly chopped

Heat a large nonstick or heavy-bottomed skillet over medium heat. Add 1 tablespoon EVOO and the onion; cook, stirring often, until softened, about 6 minutes.

Stir in sundried tomatoes, olives, and garlic and cook for 2 to 3 minutes, adding vegetable broth if too dry.

Stir in the crumbled tofu, turmeric, and oregano and season to taste; cook for about 6 to 7 minutes. Stir in the nutritional yeast and basil and turn off the heat.

Arrange avocado slices and scatter the walnuts on top of the scramble and serve immediately.

Recipe Note

- *Fold in a cup of spinach or kale at the end before serving for added nutritional boost.*

MIGHTY SMOOTHIE BOWL

FOR THE SMOOTHIE

1 ripe banana, peeled and chopped

½ cup frozen mangoes

3 kiwis, peeled and chopped

1 packed cup kale

1 teaspoon each of grated fresh turmeric and ginger (or ½ teaspoon ground)

1½ cups unsweetened almond or other plant-based milk of choice

1 tablespoon unsweetened almond or other nut butter of choice

1½ tablespoons chia seeds

1½ tablespoons flaxseeds

FOR SERVING

⅓ cup blueberries

3 tablespoons chopped walnuts

1 medium-size apple, chopped

1 sliced kiwi

1½ tablespoons cacao nibs (optional)

NEURO 9 ITEMS: kale, almond butter, chia seeds, flaxseeds, blueberries, walnuts, spices

PREP TIME: 10 minutes

COOKING TIME: none

TOTAL TIME: 10 minutes

YIELD: 3 servings

Blend all smoothie ingredients in a high-speed blender; divide equally among three serving bowls.

Scatter on top of each smoothie bowl 2 tablespoons blueberries, 1 tablespoon chopped walnuts, a third of the chopped apples, kiwi, and cacao nibs, if using. Serve immediately.

Recipe Note

• Add some monk fruit sweetener to taste.

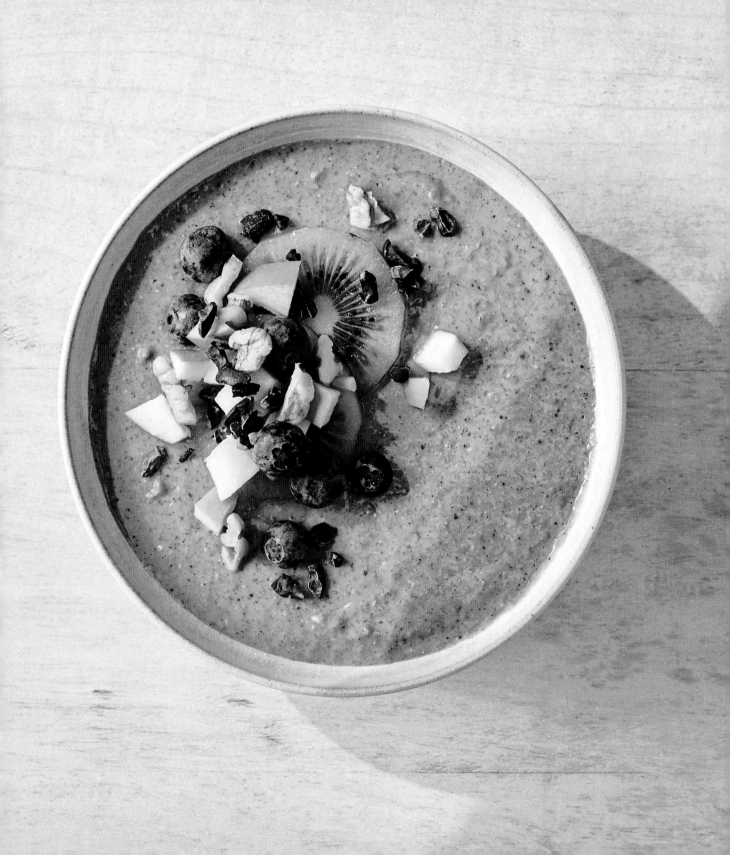

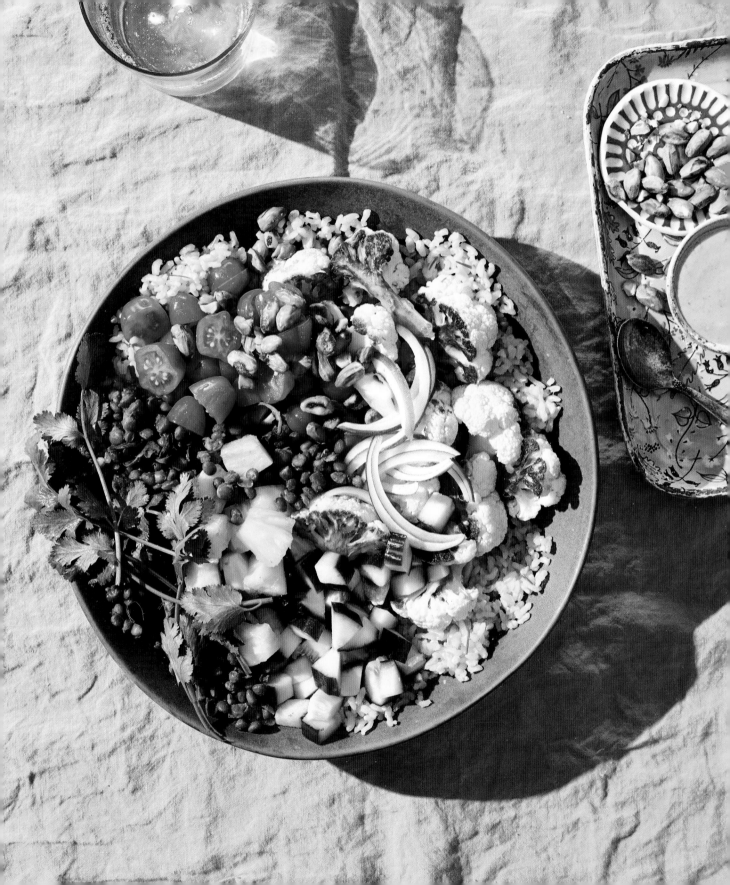

SAFFRON RICE CURRIED LENTIL BOWL

FOR THE DRESSING

¼ cup tahini

Juice and zest of 1 large lime (or to taste)

Pinch each of curry powder, ground cumin, and garlic powder

Salt and freshly ground black pepper, to taste

FOR THE BOWL

Pinch of saffron

1 teaspoon hot water

1 cup uncooked brown basmati rice

1½ teaspoons curry paste

1½ cups cooked lentils, drained

2 packed cups baby kale or baby spinach

1 cup roasted cauliflower (recipe page 175)

½ cup each of diced tomatoes and diced cucumbers

¼ cup each of diced red onion and diced fresh pineapple

2 tablespoons each of chopped cilantro and pistachios

NEURO 9 ITEMS: brown rice, lentils, kale, tahini, pistachio nuts, herbs and spices

PREP TIME: 15 minutes

COOKING TIME: 3–4 minutes

TOTAL TIME: 18–19 minutes

YIELD: 3 servings

Whisk together tahini, lime zest and juice, and spices, gradually adding enough cold water to achieve a dressing consistency. Season with salt and pepper to taste and refrigerate until needed.

Add saffron to a small bowl and crush with the back of a spoon, then mix with 1 teaspoon hot water. Add the rice and cook according to packet instructions.

Heat a large skillet over medium heat, spray with EVOO, and add curry paste; heat for about 10 seconds, until fragrant. Add the lentils and kale and cook for 3 to 4 minutes, until the kale has wilted. Season with salt and pepper to taste and remove from heat.

Fluff the rice with a fork and divide among three serving bowls. Spoon lentils and kale in the center and arrange roasted cauliflower, tomatoes, cucumber, red onion, and pineapple around. Scatter cilantro and pistachios on top and serve with the dressing on the side.

Recipe Notes

- *Substitute curry paste with 1½ teaspoons curry powder mixed with 1 tablespoon water.*

- *Add heat to the topping with sliced green chili pepper.*

- *Add a bay leaf and 2 cardamom pods to the rice to make it more aromatic.*

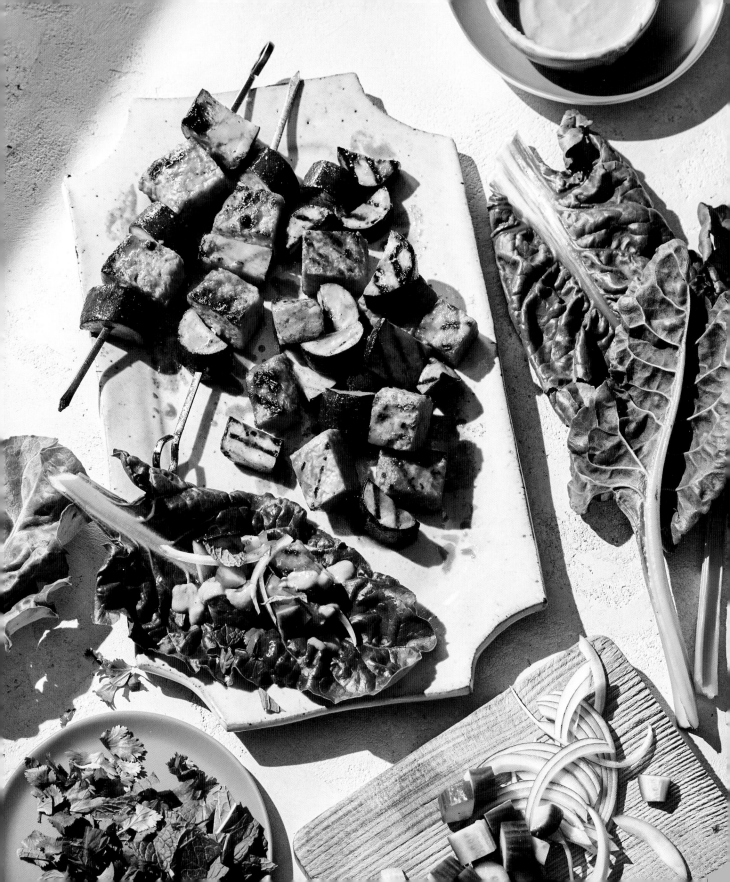

GRILLED TEMPEH SATAY WRAPS

NEURO 9 ITEMS: tempeh, peanuts (a legume), Swiss chard, spring greens, herbs and spices

PREP TIME: 10 minutes

COOKING TIME: 15 minutes

TOTAL TIME: 25 minutes

YIELD: 3 servings

FOR THE SKEWERS

2 tablespoons reduced-sodium tamari or soy sauce

EVOO spray

2 teaspoons sriracha or other chili sauce of choice (or to taste), divided

½ teaspoon each of ground turmeric and cumin

1 8-ounce package tempeh, cut into 1-inch cubes

2 medium yellow squash or zucchini, cut into 1-inch pieces

Sea salt and freshly ground black pepper, to taste

3 wooden skewers, soaked in water

FOR THE SATAY SAUCE

3 tablespoons unsalted peanut butter

½ teaspoon finely grated fresh ginger

1 garlic clove, minced

1 teaspoon liquid aminos or tamari sauce

Juice of 1 large lime (or to taste)

FOR THE WRAPS

6 large Swiss chard leaves, trimmed (or 3 100% whole-wheat wraps)

1 small red onion, thinly sliced

2 small cucumbers, cut into matchsticks

2 cups mixed baby spring greens

2 tablespoons each of chopped fresh mint and cilantro

Whisk tamari, EVOO, sriracha sauce, turmeric, and cumin in a small bowl.

Place tempeh and squash in a mixing bowl and toss with the tamari mixture, coating evenly. Season to taste with salt and pepper, and thread, alternating, onto the skewers. If time permits, let marinate for 10 to 15 minutes.

Heat a grill pan over medium heat, then reduce to medium-low. Add the skewers and grill, turning often, until golden and grill marks appear. You may need to spray the skewers with EVOO to keep them from sticking to the pan. Set aside.

Whisk all satay sauce ingredients in a small bowl until smooth, adding just enough water to get the desired consistency; adjust seasoning to taste and set aside.

Remove the grilled tempeh and squash from the skewers and divide among the Swiss chard leaves. Top with the onion, cucumbers, and baby greens and drizzle with the sauce. Scatter mint and cilantro over the filling and roll up tightly. Cut each wrap in half and serve.

FALAFEL WRAPS WITH ZA'ATAR TAHINI

FOR THE FALAFEL

1 15-ounce can chickpeas, drained

1/3 cup walnuts

2 garlic cloves, minced

1 small onion, chopped

1/2 teaspoon ground cumin

1 teaspoon coriander

1/3 cup each of cilantro, mint, and flat-leaf parsley, chopped

1/2 teaspoon baking powder

Salt and freshly ground black pepper, to taste

Avocado oil spray

FOR THE TAHINI SAUCE

1/3 cup tahini

Juice of 1 large lemon

2 teaspoons za'atar seasoning (or to taste)

Pinch of cayenne pepper

FOR THE WRAPS

3 medium 100% whole-wheat lavash flatbread

1 large cucumber, chopped

1 tomato, seeded and diced

1 red onion, sliced into moon-shaped slivers

2 cups kale, shredded and massaged for 1 minute

NEURO 9 ITEMS: chickpeas, walnuts, kale, tahini, 100% whole-wheat lavash flatbread, herbs and spices

PREP TIME: 15 minutes plus 1 hour for chilling

COOKING TIME: 20 minutes

TOTAL TIME: 35 minutes

YIELD: 3 servings

Line a baking sheet with parchment paper or a silicone baking mat and set aside.

Tip all falafel ingredients into a food processor and pulse until combined but not too smooth. If the mixture is too dry, add about a tablespoon of water. Season to taste.

Using a small ice cream scoop, shape the mixture into balls and arrange on the prepared baking sheet. Flatten into patties and refrigerate until firm (about 1 hour), or alternatively, place in freezer for about 15 minutes.

Preheat the oven to 400°F. Lightly spray the falafel with avocado oil and bake until golden (about 18 to 20 minutes), flipping over halfway though.

Meanwhile, whisk all tahini sauce ingredients with enough water to get a runny consistency, season to taste, and refrigerate until needed.

Warm the lavash bread. Place falafel, cucumber, tomatoes, red onions, and kale on bread and drizzle with the tahini sauce, then roll gently. Serve immediately.

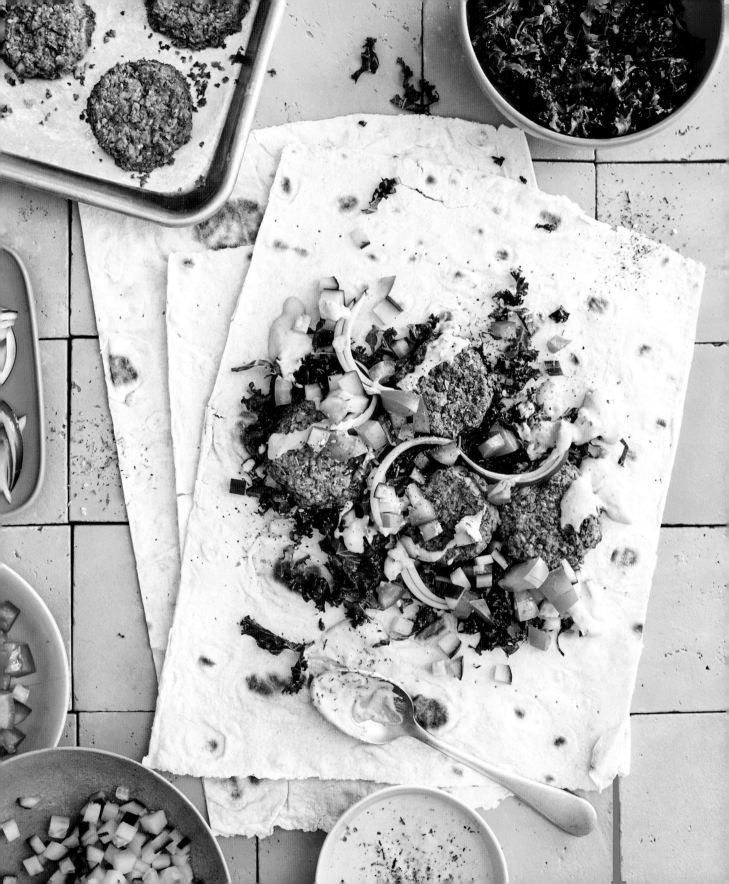

SHIITAKE CHICKPEA BULGUR BOWL

NEURO 9 ITEMS: chickpeas, kale, broccolini, bulgur wheat, tahini, herbs and spices

PREP TIME: 15 minutes

COOKING TIME: 30 minutes

TOTAL TIME: 45 minutes

YIELD: 3 servings

FOR THE BOWL

1 15.5-ounce can chickpeas, drained and rinsed

½ teaspoon each of paprika, cumin, and turmeric

1 tablespoon plus 1 teaspoon avocado oil, divided

3 cups sliced kale, stalks removed

Squeeze of lemon juice

Salt and freshly ground black pepper, to taste

3 cups shiitake mushrooms, caps only (or any kind of mushrooms)

1 bunch of broccolini

¼ cup balsamic vinegar

1 cup uncooked bulgur wheat

FOR THE DRESSING

⅓ cup tahini

Juice of 1 lemon

3 tablespoons chopped fresh herbs (e.g., dill, parsley, mint, chives)

1 large garlic clove, minced

Preheat the oven to 425°F. Line two rimmed baking sheets with parchment paper.

Carefully dry the chickpeas with a towel and place in a bowl, toss with ½ tablespoon avocado oil, spices, and salt to taste. Spread onto one of the prepared baking sheets and roast, stirring occasionally, for about 30 minutes, or until crunchy and browned.

Place kale in a large bowl, drizzle with 1 teaspoon avocado oil and a squeeze of lemon juice, season with salt, and massage with your hands until slightly wilted. Transfer to the second baking sheet and bake until crispy, about 10 minutes, tossing halfway through. Tip into a bowl and set aside.

Meanwhile, add mushrooms and broccolini to a mixing bowl and toss with remaining ½ tablespoon avocado oil and the balsamic vinegar; season with salt and pepper and set aside for 5 to 10 minutes to marinate.

Heat a grill pan over medium heat and grill the mushrooms and broccolini (in batches as needed) for about 2 to 3 minutes per side or until grill marks appear.

Cook the bulgur wheat as per packet instructions; season to taste and set aside.

In a small bowl, whisk all dressing ingredients with just enough water to get a runny consistency; adjust seasoning to taste and set aside.

Divide bulgur among three serving bowls and pile the mushrooms, broccoli, kale, and chickpeas on top. Serve drizzled with the tahini dressing.

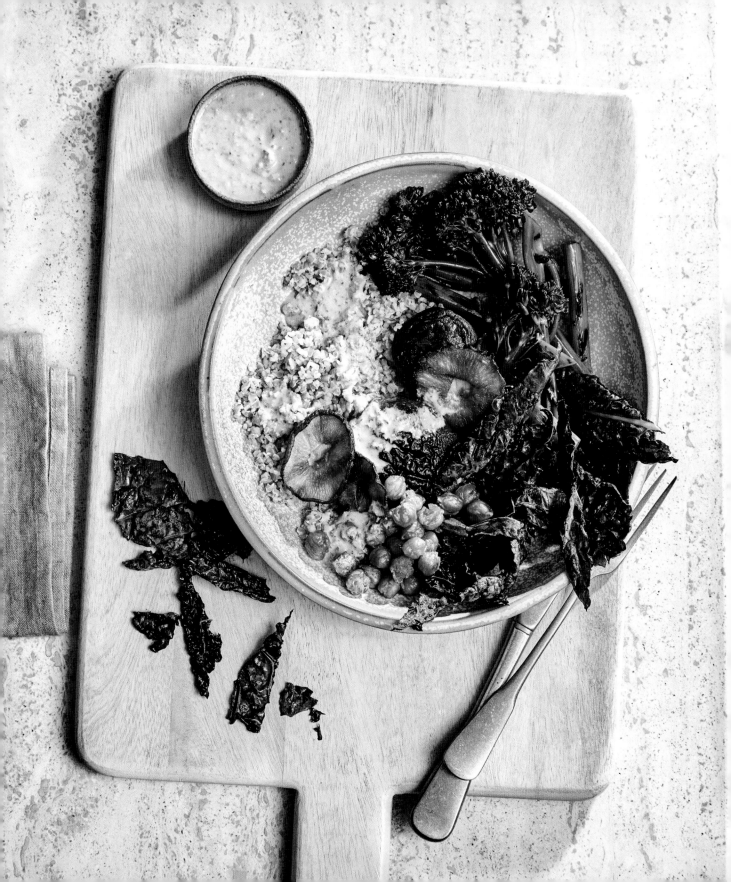

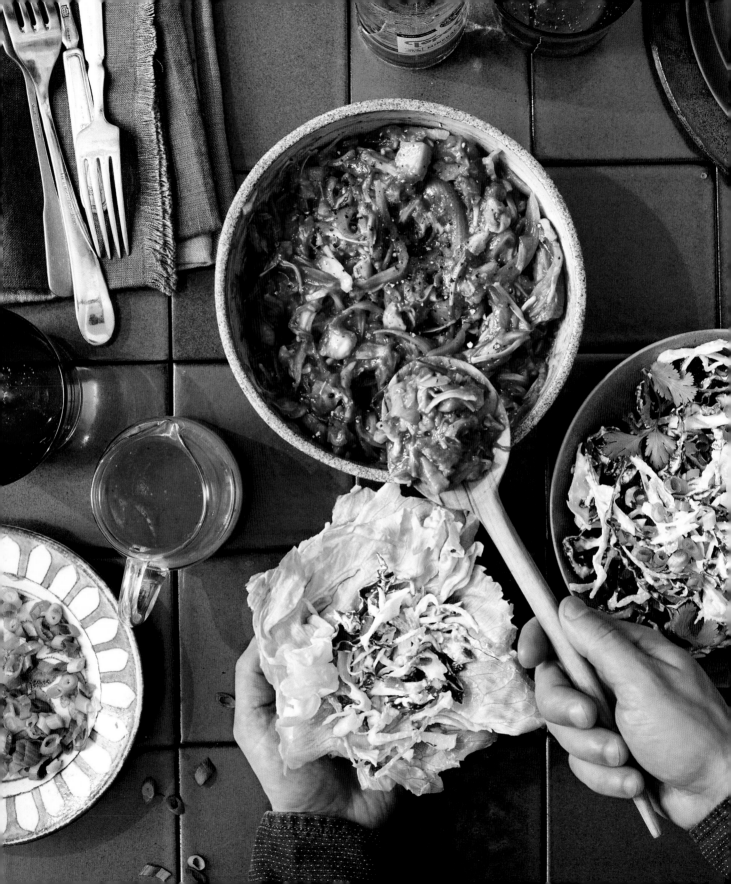

BBQ JACKFRUIT LETTUCE WRAPS

FOR THE JACKFRUIT

1 14-ounce can young green jackfruit in brine

1 tablespoon EVOO

1 small red onion, thinly sliced

2 garlic cloves, minced

½ cup low-sugar or sugar-free barbecue sauce

1 teaspoon hot sauce (or to taste)

2 tablespoons lime juice

1 teaspoon monk fruit sweetener (optional)

½ cup water or low-sodium vegetable broth

FOR THE TOFU MAYONNAISE

½ cup firm tofu, cubed

Juice of ½ lemon (or to taste)

½ teaspoon Dijon mustard

⅓ cup raw cashews, soaked in boiling water for at least 30 minutes or in room-temperature water overnight

Salt and freshly ground black pepper, to taste

FOR THE WRAPS

1 cup shredded red or green cabbage

1 red bell pepper, deseeded and finely chopped

1 jalapeño pepper, seeds and pith removed, finely chopped

1 large carrot, coarsely grated

3 scallions, finely chopped

3 tablespoons chopped cilantro or parsley

6 large iceberg lettuce leaves

NEURO 9 ITEMS: tofu, cashews, cabbage, lettuce, herbs and spices

PREP TIME: 15 minutes, not including the 30 minutes of soaking

COOKING TIME: 25 minutes

TOTAL TIME: 40 minutes

YIELD: 3 servings (2 wraps per serving)

Rinse and drain the jackfruit in a colander. Sort through the pieces of the jackfruit and separate the tough core parts from the rest. Cut them into smaller pieces and add them back to the rest of the fruit. Rinse again and pat dry with a tea towel. Heat EVOO in a skillet over medium heat and add onion and garlic; cook for about 3 to 4 minutes, then stir in jackfruit, barbecue sauce, hot sauce, lime juice, monk fruit, and water or broth. Stir to mix and bring to a boil, then reduce heat to medium-low, cover with a lid, and let simmer, stirring occasionally, until the sauce has thickened (about 25 minutes). If there is any remaining liquid, remove the lid and cook over medium heat for a few minutes.

Once the jackfruit is softened, shred it using two forks, adding more barbecue sauce, lime juice, or hot sauce to adjust to your liking.

In a blender, blend all mayonnaise ingredients, adding enough water to get the desired consistency. Season to taste and set aside.

Combine cabbage, red bell and jalapeño peppers, carrot, scallions, and cilantro in a bowl and toss with mayonnaise; adjust the seasoning if needed to taste.

Divide the jackfruit and coleslaw among the lettuce leaves, roll up, and serve with extra barbecue sauce on the side.

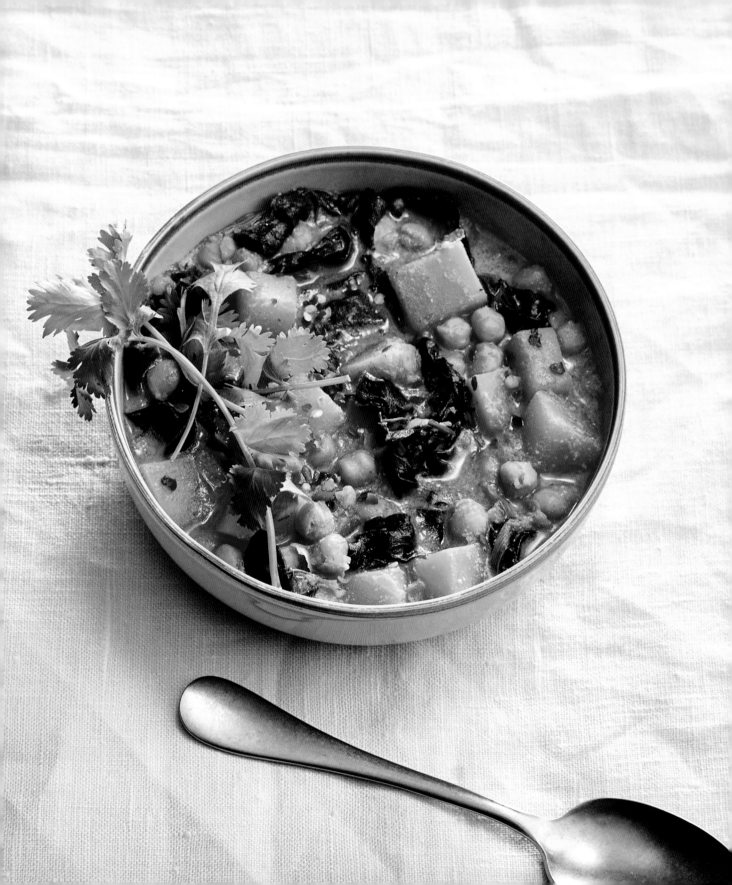

BUTTERNUT SQUASH CHICKPEA CURRY

1 teaspoon EVOO

½ medium yellow onion, chopped

3 to 4 garlic cloves, crushed

2 tablespoons finely grated fresh ginger

1 teaspoon ground turmeric

2 tablespoons yellow or red curry paste

2 cups cubed butternut squash

2 15-ounce cans chickpeas, drained and rinsed

2 cups low-sodium vegetable broth

1 tablespoon liquid aminos

½ cup raw cashews, soaked in boiling water for at least 30 minutes or in room-temperature water overnight

¾ cup water

3 cups spinach

Juice of 1 large lime

Salt and freshly ground black pepper, to taste

¼ cup each of mint leaves and cilantro, chopped

Red pepper flakes, to taste

NEURO 9 ITEMS: cashews, chickpeas, spinach, turmeric, herbs

PREP TIME: 15 minutes, not including the 30 minutes of soaking

COOKING TIME: 20 minutes

TOTAL TIME: 35 minutes plus soaking time for cashews

YIELD: 3 servings

Heat a large saucepan over medium heat, add the EVOO and onion and sauté for about 3 minutes, until soft. Add the garlic, ginger, turmeric, and curry paste, and cook for 2 to 3 minutes.

Add the butternut squash and stir. Cook for 3 minutes. Add the chickpeas, vegetable broth, and liquid aminos. Reduce the heat to medium-low, cover, and simmer until the butternut squash is just tender, about 10 minutes.

Drain the cashews and place in a blender with ¾ cup water; blend until creamy and smooth. Add a little more water if needed. Add this cashew cream to the squash mixture and bring to a quick boil. Add splashes of vegetable broth during the cooking process as needed.

Stir in the spinach and cook until wilted, about 2 minutes. Turn off the heat and add lime juice; adjust salt and pepper as needed.

Top with mint and cilantro leaves and garnish with lime wedges. Serve with quinoa or brown rice. Add a few broccoli florets to make it more nutritious.

PINTO BEAN QUESADILLA WITH CHIPOTLE CASHEW QUESO

NEURO 9 ITEMS: pinto beans, cashews, spinach, red cabbage, 100% whole-grain tortilla, spices

PREP TIME: 15 minutes

COOKING TIME: 20 minutes

TOTAL TIME: 35 minutes

YIELD: 6 servings

EVOO spray

1 red or green bell pepper, diced

½ cup frozen or fresh corn

1 15-ounce can no salt added pinto beans, drained

¼ teaspoon cumin

¼ teaspoon black pepper

1 cup Chipotle Cashew Queso, divided (page 205)

1 cup spinach leaves, chopped

2 cups shredded red cabbage

6 sprouted whole-grain tortillas, or 100% whole-wheat tortillas

Cilantro, chopped, for garnish

Heat a nonstick pan over medium heat. Spray with EVOO and add bell pepper and corn; sauté for 2 minutes (if the corn is frozen, sauté a bit longer). Mash at least half of the pinto beans with the back of a wooden spoon or fork and add to the pan. Add the cumin and the black pepper and stir.

Add ½ cup Chipotle Cashew Queso and stir. When warm, fold in the spinach and red cabbage and turn off the heat.

To make a quesadilla, place a tortilla on a nonstick pan over medium heat. Warm on one side for 15 seconds and flip to the other side. Spread 3 to 4 spoonfuls of the filling over half the tortilla (about a half inch of filling). Drizzle a little of the remaining queso over the tortilla and fold it in half to make a half moon–shaped quesadilla. Flip it over in the pan so that both sides are crispy.

Remove from the pan. Make five more quesadillas, or until you are out of filling. Cut each quesadilla into three wedges and serve warm with more queso, guacamole, or salsa.

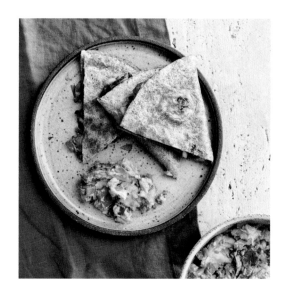

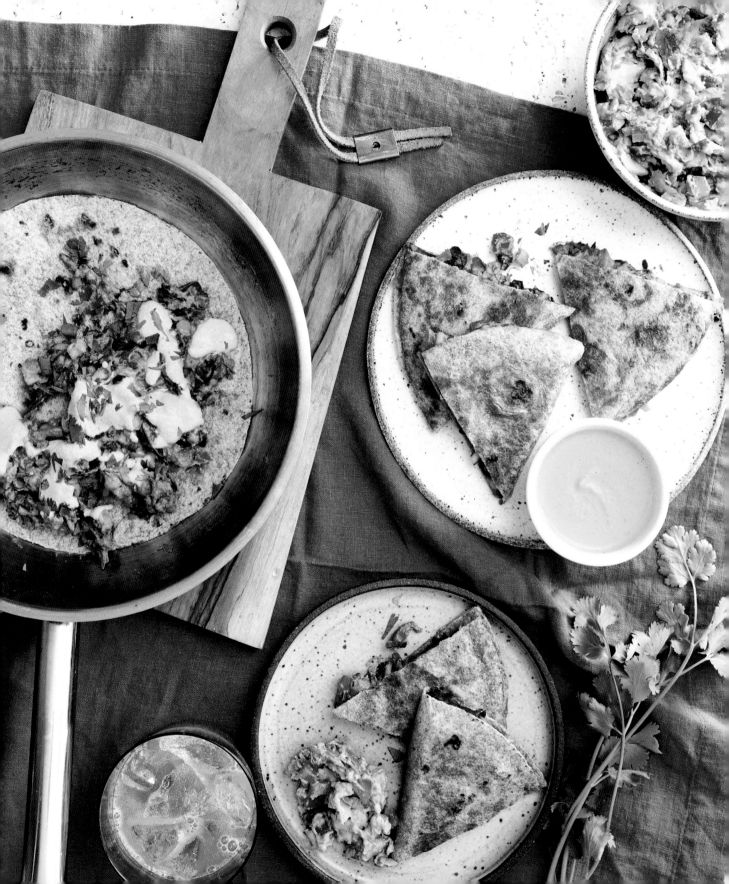

TOTALLY POSSIBLE BURGERS

EVOO spray

2 cups chopped cremini mushrooms

½ cup walnuts

1 cup rolled oats

1 teaspoon tapioca flour

1 15-ounce can black beans

1 15-ounce can chickpeas

1½ cups cooked lentils or 1 15-ounce can lentils

3 tablespoons nutritional yeast

1 teaspoon liquid smoke (optional)

2 teaspoons liquid aminos

¼ teaspoon black pepper

½ to 1 teaspoon red chili flakes for heat (optional)

1 small beet, peeled and shredded

Salt, to taste

½ cup parsley leaves, chopped

100% whole-wheat buns, preferably sprouted

1 tablespoon Chipotle Cashew Queso (page 205)

OPTIONAL GARNISHES

Sliced cucumbers, onion slices, butter lettuce leaves, and pickled jalapeños

NEURO 9 ITEMS: walnuts, oats, beans (black beans, chickpeas, lentils), butter lettuce, 100% sprouted whole-wheat buns, herbs and spices

PREP TIME: 15 minutes plus 20 minutes freezer time

COOKING TIME: 35 minutes

TOTAL TIME: 70 minutes

YIELD: 4 servings

Heat a large nonstick skillet on high. Spray the surface of the pan with a little bit of EVOO. Then add the mushrooms and cook for about 10 minutes so they lose their moisture. Set aside.

Add the walnuts to a blender or food processor and pulse to create a walnut meal (very finely processed but not so much so that it becomes walnut butter). Then add the oats and tapioca flour and pulse three to four times to pulverize the oats slightly. You don't want to create oat flour; just break it down so it's smaller in texture. It's fine if there are some large oat pieces left. Add the black beans, chickpeas, half of the lentils, nutritional yeast, liquid smoke, liquid aminos, black pepper, and chili flakes, if using, to the processor. Gently pulse all the ingredients to create a mostly ground mixture. Then add the beet and pulse until the ingredients begin to come together.

Transfer the mixture to a mixing bowl. Adjust salt and heat to taste. Add chopped parsley and mix. Shape into four to six patties. Line a baking sheet with parchment paper and place the patties on the baking sheet and chill in the fridge for 15 to 20 minutes.

Preheat the oven to 375°F. While it's warming, heat a nonstick pan on high heat and spray with EVOO. Arrange the chilled patties on the pan and sauté for about 10 minutes on one side until browned, then flip and continue sautéing for another 10 minutes. Place the burgers on the lined baking sheet and bake in the heated oven for 15 minutes until browned and firm.

ARRANGE THE BURGER: Toast the 100% sprouted whole-wheat buns. Spread a little Chipotle Cashew Queso on half of a bun and then place desired toppings like onions, tomatoes, and lettuce; place a patty on top of them and spread on more queso. Then top with the other half of the bun.

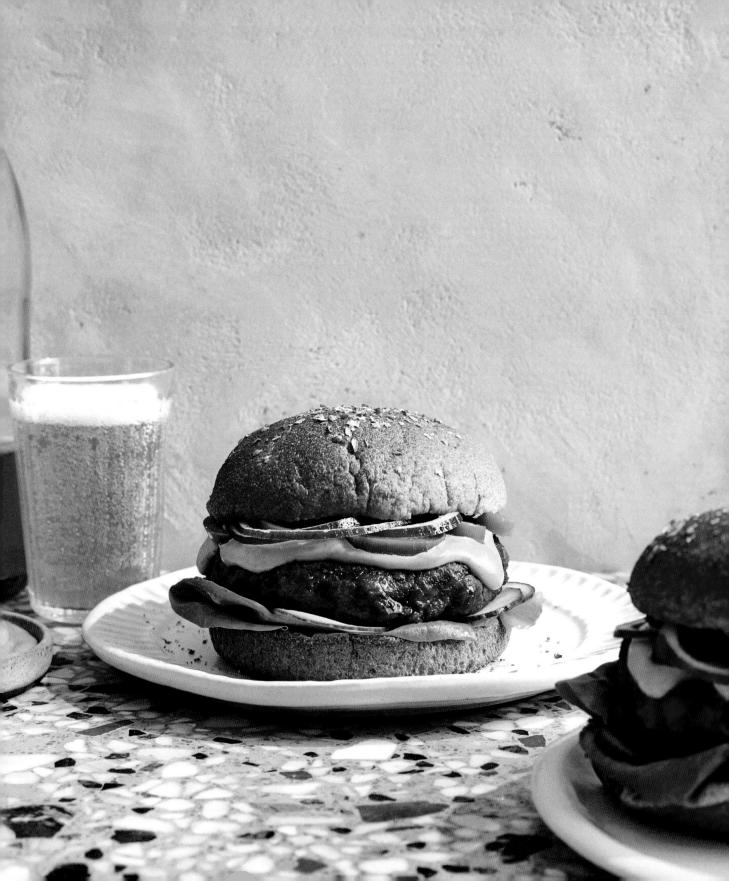

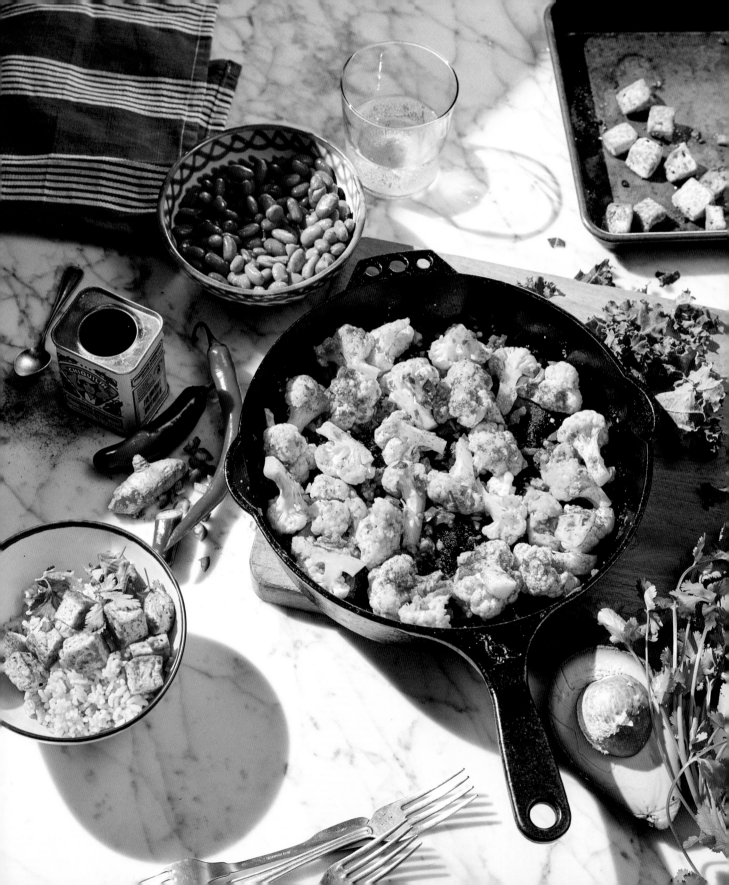

SPICY CAULI TOFU BOWL

Avocado oil spray

1 14-ounce block tofu, pressed, drained and cut into 1-inch cubes

1 teaspoon each of cumin and smoked paprika, divided

Salt and peper, to taste

1 teaspoon each of cumin and smoked paprika

1 red or green chili pepper, chopped

1 teaspoon each of finely grated fresh ginger and fresh turmeric

2 garlic cloves, crushed

2 cups cauliflower or broccoli florets

1 bunch of at least 4 cups curly kale, tough stems removed and thinly sliced

1 15.5-ounce can no salt added pinto beans, drained and rinsed

2 cups cooked brown rice

OPTIONAL GARNISHES

1 ripe avocado, sliced

Juice and zest of 1 lemon

Crushed red pepper

Small handful cilantro, chopped

NEURO 9 ITEMS: kale, tofu, brown rice, cauliflower, pinto beans, herbs

PREP TIME: 15 minutes

COOKING TIME: 25 minutes

TOTAL TIME: 35–40 minutes

YIELD: 4 servings

Place tofu in a bowl and sprinkle with ½ teaspoon cumin and ½ teaspoon paprika; season with salt and pepper to taste, toss gently, and set aside.

Heat a spray or two of avocado oil in a large skillet over medium heat and stir in chili pepper, ginger, turmeric, and garlic. Stir for 1minute until fragrant. Add cauliflower, ½ teaspoon paprika, ½ teaspoon cumin, and a pinch of salt, and cover with a lid. Reduce heat to medium-low, add 2 tablespoons of water and cook, stirring occasionally, until the cauliflower is just tender, about 10 minutes. Using a slotted spoon, transfer to a plate and keep warm.

Add kale and pinto beans to the skillet and cook, stirring often, for about 3 minutes, or until beans are heated through and kale has wilted. If needed, add a tablespoon of vegetable broth as you cook to prevent the mixture from getting too dry.

Set the broiler to high. Line a small baking sheet with a silicone baking mat or parchment paper and arrange tofu on top. Spray with avocado oil. Cook for about 4 to 5 minutes, then turn the pieces and let cook for another 5 minutes until the tofu is browned.

Divide brown rice among four bowls and top with cauliflower, beans, kale, and tofu. Garnish with sliced avocado, lemon juice, and crushed red pepper and sprinkle with chopped cilantro before serving.

Recipe Note

- *Drizzle with Almond Chipotle Sauce (page 209).*

CREAMY MUSHROOM AND RADICCHIO PASTA BAKE

1 8-ounce box whole-wheat penne pasta (or brown rice or lentil pasta)

EVOO spray

1 small red onion, chopped

2 garlic cloves, crushed

2 cups cremini mushrooms, sliced

2 heads (each about 4 ounces) red radicchio, thinly sliced

Leaves from 2 sprigs of fresh thyme

1 bunch of Swiss chard, tough stems removed and leaves thinly sliced

Salt and freshly ground black pepper, to taste

¼ cup whole-grain breadcrumbs

FOR THE SAUCE

4 tablespoons 100% whole-wheat flour

3 cups unsweetened almond milk, divided

2 tablespoons tahini

¼ cup nutritional yeast

Generous pinch of ground nutmeg

½ teaspoon each of salt and freshly ground black pepper, to taste

NEURO 9 ITEMS: radicchio, Swiss chard, tahini, thyme, nutmeg

PREP TIME: 15 minutes

COOKING TIME: 40 minutes

TOTAL TIME: 55 minutes

YIELD: 4 servings

In a large pot, cook pasta according to the package directions; drain well and return to the pot; set aside.

Preheat the oven to 400°F. Lightly spray a 7-by-10.5-inch rectangular baking dish with EVOO spray.

Heat a large heavy-bottomed skillet over medium heat and spray with EVOO. Sauté onions for a few minutes or until softened, then add garlic and mushrooms. Cook until the mushrooms are tender and most of the liquid has evaporated, about 8 to 10 minutes. Then add the radicchio, thyme leaves, and Swiss chard and cook until wilted, about 2 minutes. Season with salt and pepper.

Mix the vegetables with the pasta and tip into the prepared baking dish. Adjust seasoning.

Whisk whole-wheat flour with a few tablespoons of almond milk in a saucepan. Once blended, slowly whisk in the remaining almond milk. Bring to a boil, then reduce the heat to medium-low and let the sauce simmer, stirring often, until thickened, 4 to 5 minutes. Stir in the tahini, nutritional yeast, and nutmeg and season to taste.

Pour the sauce on top of the pasta and vegetables, then sprinkle with breadcrumbs. Bake for 20 to 25 minutes, or until the sauce is bubbling and the top is lightly browned. Serve immediately. Leftovers keep in an airtight container for a couple of days in the refrigerator.

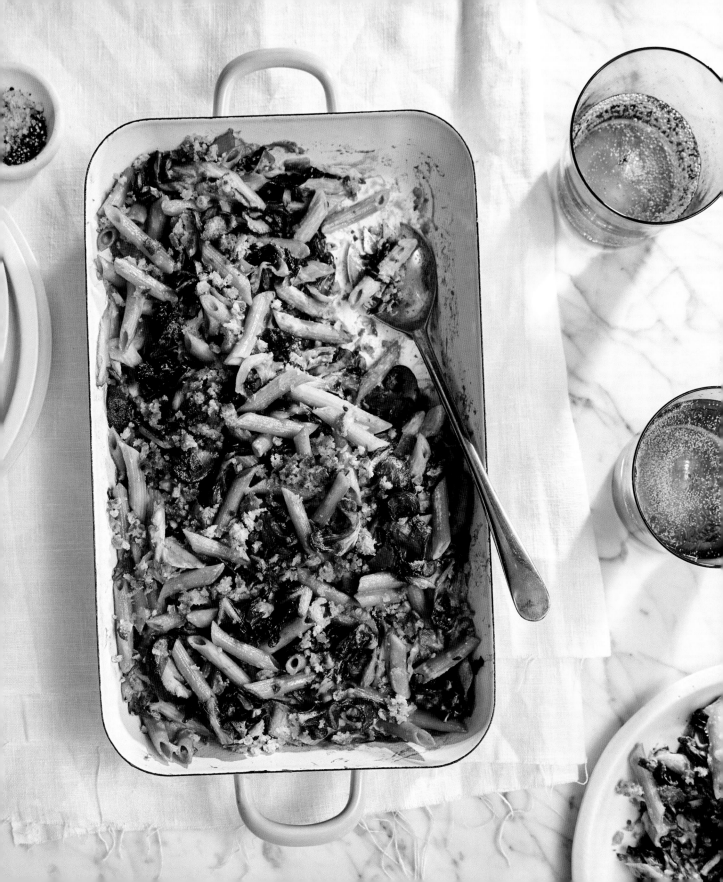

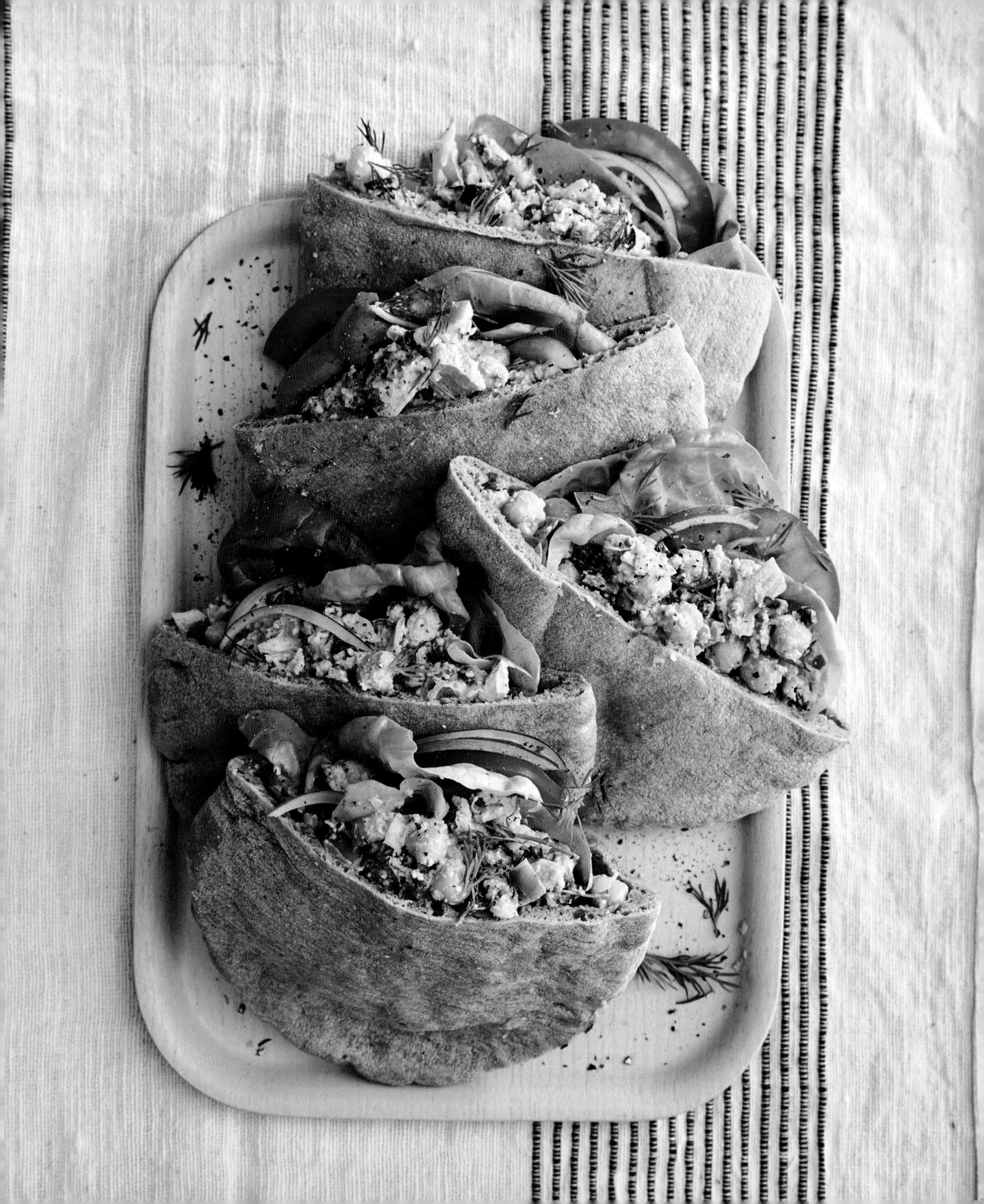

CHICKPEA AND SEEDS SANDWICH

FOR THE SALAD

½ cup raw sunflower seeds, soaked in boiling water for 30 minutes or in room-temperature water overnight, drained and rinsed

3 tablespoons tahini

1 tablespoon liquid aminos

1 teaspoon Dijon mustard

2 tablespoons nutritional yeast

3 tablespoons lemon juice

1 cup canned no salt added chickpeas, rinsed and drained

¼ cup of each of chopped red onion and celery (half a small red onion and 1 large stalk of celery)

1 tablespoon capers, drained and chopped (optional)

2 tablespoons chopped fresh dill or fennel fronds

Sea salt and freshly ground black pepper, to taste

TO ASSEMBLE

4 medium 100% whole-wheat pita breads

OPTIONAL GARNISHES

Sliced red onion, cucumber, tomato, avocado, and lettuce

NEURO 9 ITEMS: sunflower seeds, tahini, chickpeas, and herbs

PREP TIME: 20 minutes

COOKING TIME: none

TOTAL TIME: 20 minutes plus soaking time for seeds

YIELD: 4 servings

Pulse sunflower seeds, tahini, liquid aminos, mustard, nutritional yeast, and lemon juice in a food processor to a coarse paste.

Mash chickpeas with a potato masher or fork in a mixing bowl, then mix with the red onion, celery, capers, if using, and dill; add the sunflower seed mixture and stir lightly to combine. Season to taste with salt and pepper.

Cut pita breads in half and fill each with 3 tablespoons of the salad mixture, adding some greens, onion slices, tomatoes, and any other desired garnishes. Serve immediately or wrap with parchment paper for later.

Recipe Note

- *Refrigerate any leftover mixture in an airtight container and use within two days.*

CAULIFLOWER CRUST PIZZA WITH TOFU RICOTTA AND ARUGULA PESTO

FOR THE PESTO

½ cup frozen peas

1 packed cup baby arugula

2 tablespoons nutritional yeast

¼ cup walnuts

2 garlic cloves

Juice of ½ lemon

3 tablespoons water
(as needed)

⅛ teaspoon salt

FOR THE TOFU RICOTTA

1 14-ounce block extra-firm tofu, drained and pressed

2 tablespoons nutritional yeast

1 garlic clove

2 teaspoons Italian herb mix or dried basil

Juice of ½ lemon

⅛ teaspoon salt

FOR THE PIZZA CRUST

4 packed cups riced cauliflower

2 tablespoons ground flaxseed mixed with ¼ cup water

2 tablespoons nutritional yeast

1½ teaspoons Italian herb mix or dried basil

2 cloves garlic, minced

1½ tablespoons cornstarch or arrowroot

Salt and freshly ground black pepper, to taste

OPTIONAL GARNISHES

Red pepper flakes

Sliced basil leaves

NEURO 9 ITEMS: peas, arugula, walnuts, tofu, cauliflower, flaxseeds, herbs and spices

PREP TIME: 15 minutes

COOKING TIME: 45–50 minutes

TOTAL TIME: 1 hour

YIELD: 6 servings

Add all the pesto ingredients to a food processor and blend until smooth, adding some water to get the desired consistency.

Add the tofu ricotta ingredients to the food processor. Pulse to mix everything and get a ricotta cheese consistency.

Preheat the oven to 400°F and line a large baking sheet with parchment paper or a silicone baking mat; set aside. If you're using a pizza stone, place it inside the oven to warm up.

In a medium pot, boil water and add the riced cauliflower. Cook for 5 minutes. Drain through a colander and spread onto a kitchen towel; set aside for a few minutes to cool. Then twist the towel and squeeze out as much moisture as possible.

Transfer the riced cauliflower to a large bowl and stir in the remaining crust ingredients and make a loose dough; season to taste.

Pile up the cauliflower mix into the center of the prepared baking sheet or a round piece of parchment paper (to be placed on top of the pizza stone or baking sheet) and spread it out with your hands to make a crust about ½-inch thick, making it slightly thicker around the edges. Bake for about 30 minutes, or until firm and golden brown.

Spread a thin layer of pesto on crust, then scatter tofu ricotta on top. Return to the oven and bake for about 10 to 12 minutes. Garnish with basil and crushed red pepper.

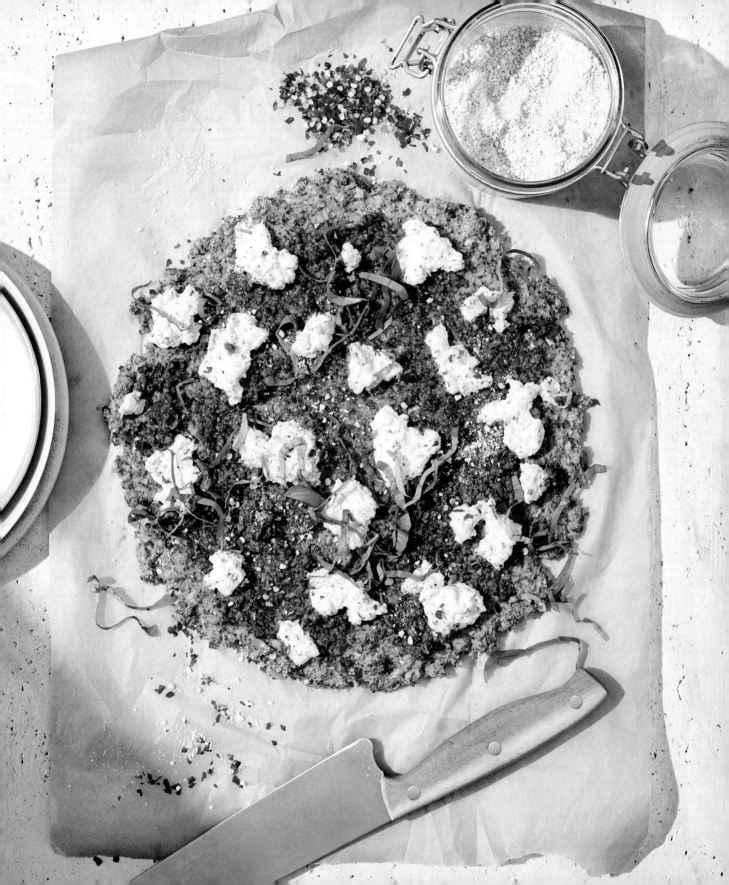

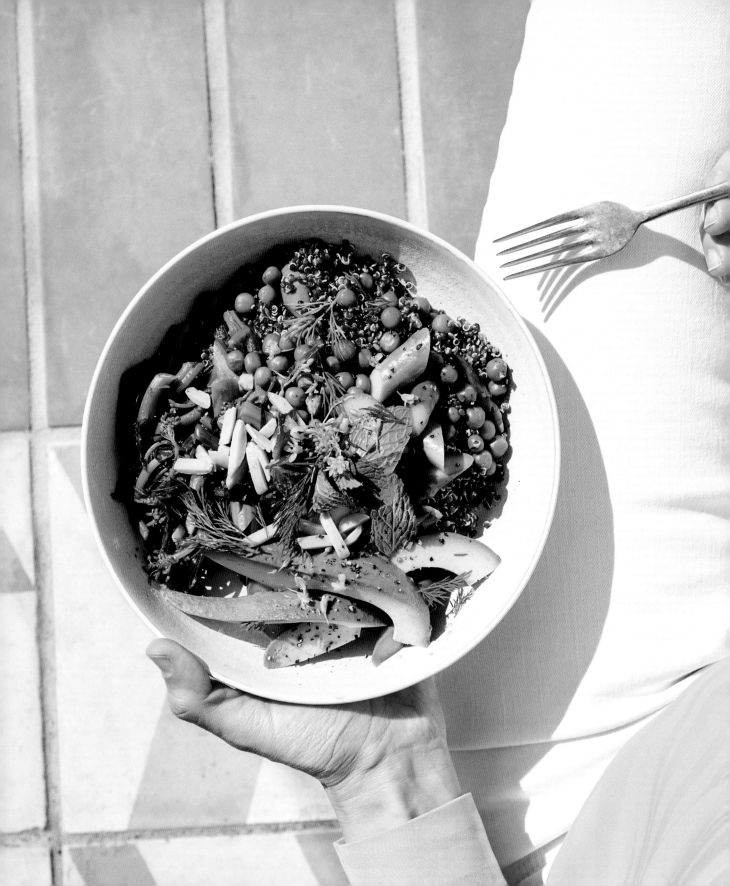

GREENS AND GRAINS POWER BOWL

¼ cup water

1 bunch (about 1 pound) of broccoli rabe, trimmed, cut into bite-size pieces, and steamed (or use 1 pound broccoli florets)

6 stalks asparagus, trimmed, cut into bite-size pieces, and steamed

1 cup cooked peas (if using frozen, steam them first)

1½ cups cooked quinoa

⅓ cup chopped mixed fresh herbs (mint, dill, and flat-leaf parsley work well)

1 ripe avocado, sliced

¼ cup toasted slivered almonds

FOR THE DRESSING

5 tablespoons unsalted almond butter

¼ teaspoon each of ground ginger and red pepper flakes

Juice of 1 large orange

Pinch of salt and pepper, to taste

NEURO 9 ITEMS: quinoa, broccoli rabe, peas, almonds, herbs

PREP TIME: 15 minutes

COOKING TIME: 5 minutes

TOTAL TIME: 20 minutes

YIELD: 3 servings

Place a pan over medium-high heat and add ¼ cup water and then add the broccoli rabe, asparagus, and peas. Cover with a lid and steam for about 5 minutes. Remove lid and let the water evaporate.

For the dressing, whisk together almond butter, ground ginger, pepper flakes, and orange juice in a small bowl until smooth; season to taste.

Combine quinoa and herbs in a bowl and toss with half of the dressing. Divide equally among three bowls and top with broccoli rabe, asparagus, peas, and avocado. Drizzle the remaining dressing on top, sprinkle with almonds, and serve.

ASIAN LETTUCE BOATS WITH MUSHROOMS

FOR THE DRESSING

Juice of ½ orange

2 tablespoons coconut aminos or reduced-sodium tamari

1 teaspoon finely grated ginger

½ tablespoon rice vinegar or apple cider vinegar

1 teaspoon sriracha or other hot sauce of choice (or to taste)

2 tablespoons unsalted peanut butter or tahini

FOR THE WRAPS

EVOO spray

1 medium onion, thinly sliced

1 celery stalk, diced

2 garlic cloves, thinly sliced

3 cups portobello mushroom caps, thinly sliced

Freshly ground black pepper, to taste

6 to 9 Bibb or Boston lettuce leaves (depending on size)

1 large carrot, cut into matchsticks

½ English cucumber, cut into matchsticks or sliced

NEURO 9 ITEMS: peanut butter or tahini, spices, lettuce

PREP TIME: 10 minutes

COOKING TIME: 15–20 minutes

TOTAL TIME: 25–30 minutes

YIELD: 3 servings (2 to 3 wraps per person)

Whisk all dressing ingredients until well-combined and refrigerate until ready to serve.

Spray a large skillet or wok with EVOO over medium heat and sauté onions and celery until softened, 2 to 3 minutes. Add garlic and mushrooms and cook, stirring frequently, until mushrooms are tender and moisture has evaporated (about 6 to 7 minutes). Add the dressing and reduce heat to low; cook, stirring often, until the sauce has thickened and the mushrooms are coated, about 7 to 10 minutes. Add pepper to taste.

Divide the mushroom mixture among the lettuce leaves, top with carrots and cucumber, and serve.

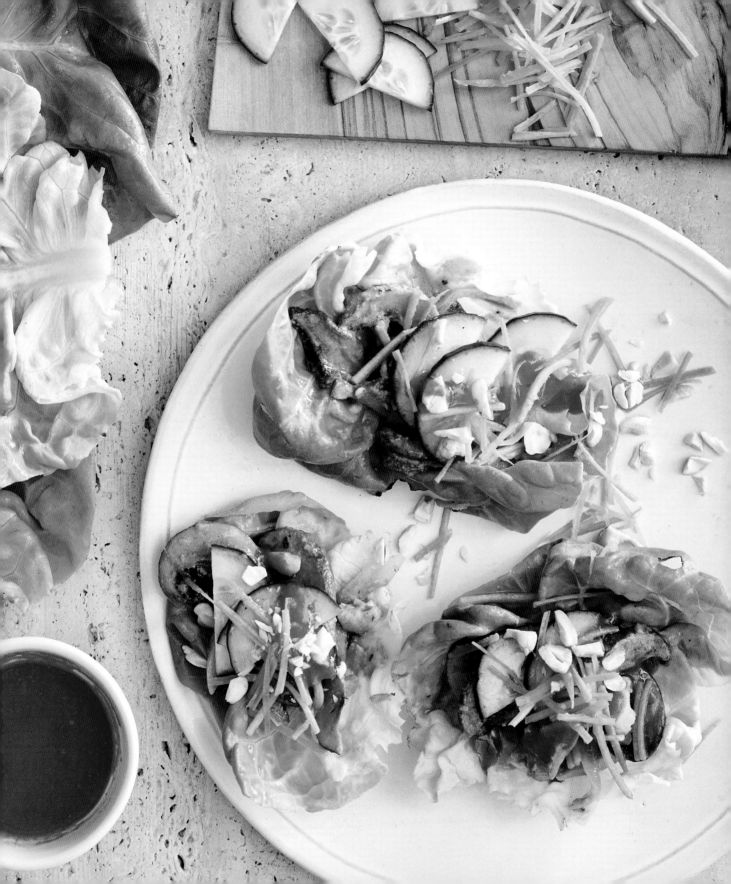

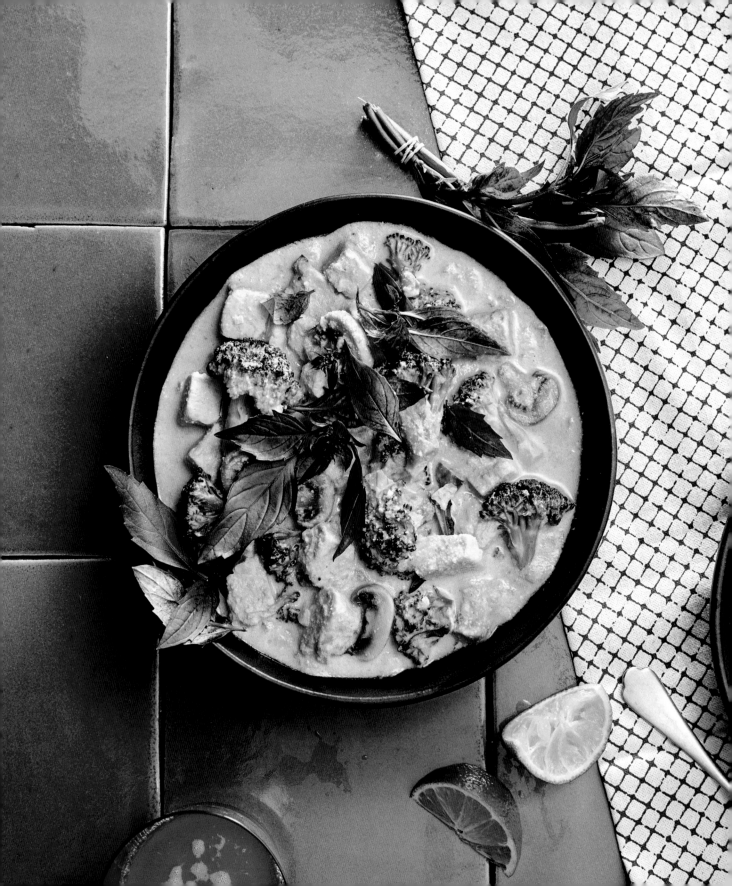

THAI TEMPEH GREEN CURRY

1 teaspoon EVOO

½ medium yellow onion, chopped

3 garlic cloves, crushed

2 tablespoons finely grated fresh ginger

1 green chili pepper, chopped

1 8-ounce block tempeh, cut into ½-inch cubes

1½ tablespoons Thai green curry paste

2 cups broccoli, cut into small florets

1 cup mushrooms, sliced

2 cups low-sodium vegetable broth, plus more as needed

½ cup raw cashews, soaked in boiling water for at least 30 minutes or in room-temperature water overnight

Juice of 1 lime

¼ cup water

Salt and freshly ground black pepper, to taste

Handful of Thai basil leaves, shredded

NEURO 9 ITEMS: cashews, tempeh, broccoli, herbs and spices

PREP TIME: 10 minutes, not including the 30 minutes of soaking

COOKING TIME: 15–20 minutes

TOTAL TIME: 25–30 minutes

YIELD: 3 servings

Heat a large saucepan over medium heat, add the EVOO and the onion, and sauté for about 3 minutes, until soft. Add the garlic, ginger, chili pepper, tempeh, and curry paste and cook for 2 minutes.

Add the broccoli and mushrooms and cook for 2 to 3 minutes, then pour in the vegetable broth and bring to a simmer.

Meanwhile, drain the cashews and place in a blender with ¼ cup water and blend until creamy and smooth. Add a little more water if needed. Add this cashew cream to the tempeh mixture and bring to a quick boil. Add splashes of the vegetable broth during the cooking process as needed. Simmer for 10 minutes or until the vegetables are tender. Add more broth if the curry looks dry.

Turn off heat and add lime juice. Season with salt and pepper as needed.

Scatter shredded basil leaves over the curry and serve.

FARRO TEMPEH BOWL

NEURO 9 ITEMS: tempeh, broccoli, kale, farro or quinoa

PREP TIME: 10 minutes

COOKING TIME: 25 minutes

TOTAL TIME: 35 minutes

YIELD: 3 servings

FOR THE TEMPEH

2 tablespoons liquid aminos

2 tablespoons balsamic vinegar

1 teaspoon adobo sauce (or to taste)

4 ounces tempeh, thinly sliced

Salt and freshly ground pepper, to taste

FOR THE BOWL

EVOO spray

1 medium sweet potato, peeled and sliced about ½-inch thick

Salt and freshly ground black pepper, to taste

1 garlic clove, minced

2 cups broccoli florets

3 cups shredded kale, stems removed

⅓ cup low-sodium vegetable broth, or as needed

1½ cups cooked farro or other grain of choice (e.g., quinoa)

1½ tablespoons nutritional yeast

1 large avocado, sliced

⅔ cup cherry or grape tomatoes, halved

Whisk liquid aminos, balsamic vinegar, and adobo sauce in a small bowl and drizzle over the tempeh slices, turning to coat well; season with salt and pepper to taste and let marinate for 10 to 15 minutes.

Heat a large nonstick skillet over medium-high heat and lightly spray with EVOO cooking spray (or add 2 tablespoons vegetable broth). Place the marinated tempeh slices in the skillet and sauté until crispy, about 8 to 10 minutes, flipping halfway through. Transfer to a plate and keep warm.

Lightly spray the same skillet with EVOO. Arrange the sweet potato slices in a single layer, season with salt and pepper, and cook for 4 to 5 minutes; then flip over and continue cooking for 5 minutes longer or until fully cooked and beginning to brown. You may need to add a splash of vegetable broth to keep the sweet potatoes from sticking to the skillet. Transfer to a plate and keep warm.

Add garlic, broccoli, kale, and 2 tablespoons broth to the skillet and season to taste. Cover with a lid and cook for about 5 minutes or until the vegetables are just tender (or cooked to your taste). Stir in the farro and nutritional yeast and heat through.

Divide the farro mixture among three serving bowls and top with tempeh, sweet potato, avocado slices, and cherry tomatoes. Serve immediately.

Recipe Notes

- *Always make sure to cook a batch of whole grains on your food prep day to have ready for the week.*

- *For more flavor, marinate tempeh overnight; you can refrigerate it for up to two days.*

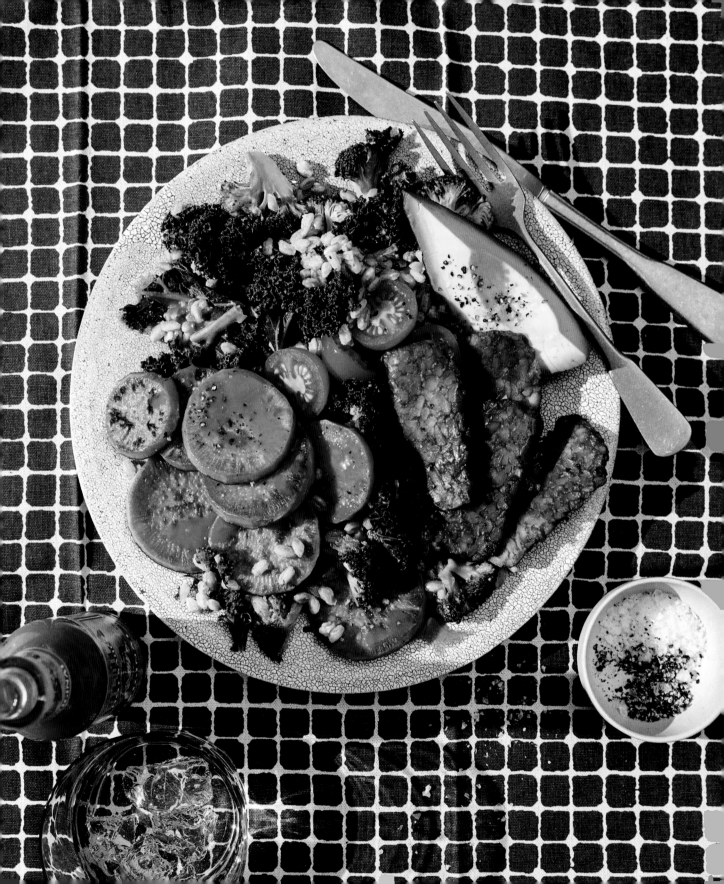

TEMPEH VEGGIE SKEWERS WITH CHIMICHURRI SAUCE

FOR THE SKEWERS

1 8-ounce package tempeh, cut into 1-inch cubes

Freshly ground black pepper, to taste

2 medium bell peppers (any color), cut into 1-inch pieces

1 medium yellow onion, cut into 1-inch pieces

1 zucchini, cut into 1-inch chunks

1 cup white button or cremini mushrooms (halved if large)

1 cup cherry tomatoes

Avocado oil spray

FOR THE CHIMICHURRI SAUCE

½ packed cup each of cilantro and flat-leaf parsley, chopped

1 large garlic clove, minced

1 red or green chili pepper, deseeded and finely chopped

1 tablespoon red wine vinegar (or to taste)

2 tablespoons lemon juice

Salt and freshly ground black pepper, to taste

1½ tablespoons EVOO

NEURO 9 ITEMS: tempeh, herbs and spices

PREP TIME: 65 minutes

COOKING TIME: 12–15 minutes

TOTAL TIME: 77–80 minutes

YIELD: 3 servings (2 skewers per serving)

6 bamboo skewers

FOR THE MARINADE

1 teaspoon spicy brown mustard

Zest and juice of 1 lime

3 tablespoons balsamic vinegar

3 tablespoons liquid aminos

3 garlic cloves, minced

2 tablespoons finely minced fresh parsley or oregano

Pinch of chili pepper or chili powder

¼ teaspoon each of salt and pepper

Place the skewers in a shallow container and cover with water; set aside.

Whisk together the marinade ingredients. Place tempeh in a mixing bowl and drizzle with the marinade; season to taste and toss to cover, then set aside for at least 1 hour, preferably 2 hours.

Heat up a grill (or preheat a broiler) to medium-high.

Thread tempeh, alternating with the vegetables, onto the skewers; reserve any leftover marinade. Spray the skewers lightly with avocado oil and grill (or broil) for about 12 to 15 minutes, flipping halfway, until the vegetables are tender and grill marks appear. If needed, brush the skewers with some of the reserved marinade during the grilling process.

Whisk the chimichurri sauce ingredients in a small bowl, adding a little water as needed; season to taste. Serve the skewers drizzled with the chimichurri sauce. Refrigerate any leftover sauce in an airtight container for up to three days.

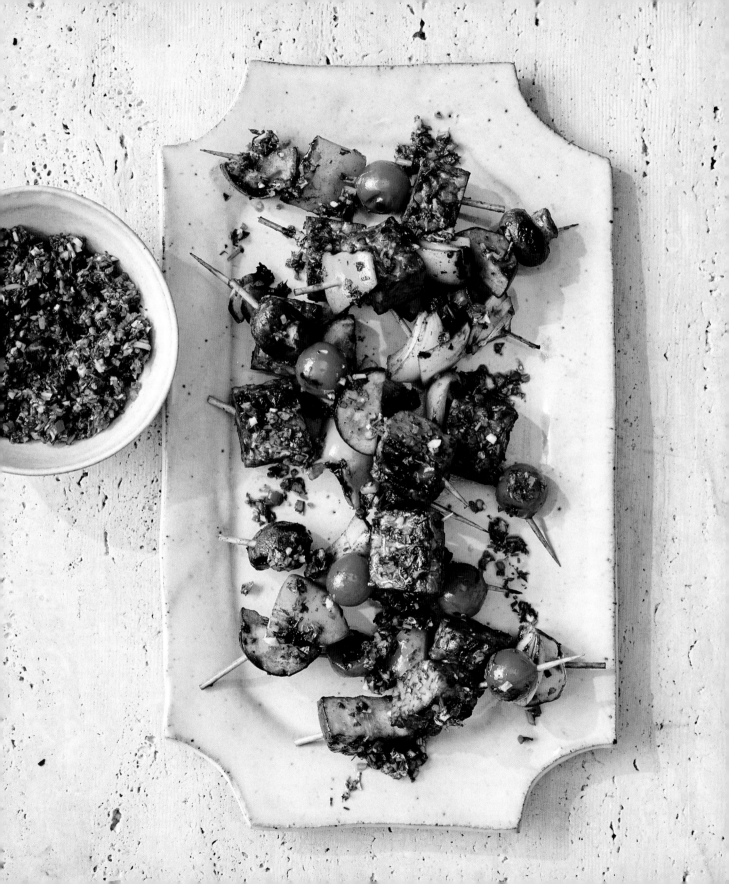

SWEET POTATO BEAN BURGER

NEURO 9 ITEMS: flaxseeds, oats, black beans, herbs and spices

PREP TIME: 15 minutes

COOKING TIME: 30 minutes

TOTAL TIME: 45 minutes

YIELD: 4 servings

2 medium sweet potatoes

1 tablespoon ground flaxseeds

3 tablespoons water

Zest and juice of 1 lime

1 teaspoon ground cumin

1 teaspoon smoked paprika

1 small red onion, finely chopped

1 jalapeño, seeds and pith removed, finely chopped

2 garlic cloves, crushed

1 tablespoon chipotle adobo sauce (not the pepper)

2/3 cup rolled oats

1 cup canned no salt added black beans, rinsed and drained

4 tablespoons chopped cilantro

Salt and freshly ground black pepper, to taste

Oat flour or cornmeal, to dust

OPTIONAL GARNISHES

Tomatoes, sliced

Avocado, sliced

Pickles, sliced

Pierce the sweet potatoes with a fork and microwave on high until tender (7 to 10 minutes), turning over halfway. Scoop out the flesh, mash roughly, and set aside to cool. Alternatively, steam or roast the sweet potatoes.

Mix flaxseeds with the water in a small bowl and let the mixture thicken, 4 to 5 minutes.

Place lime zest and juice, cumin, paprika, onion, jalapeño, garlic, chipotle sauce, and oats in a food processor and pulse until ingredients begin to come together. Add black beans and cilantro, season to taste, and pulse a few times to incorporate.

Transfer the mixture to a mixing bowl and shape into four patties with wet hands, as mixture will be sticky. Dust the patties with some oat flour and place in the freezer for 10 to 15 minutes.

Preheat the oven to 400°F and line a baking sheet with parchment paper or a silicone baking mat. Arrange the chilled patties on the prepared baking sheet and bake for about 15 minutes, then flip over and continue baking for another 5 minutes.

Recipe Notes

- *Serve on a sprouted whole-wheat bun or on a bed of greens with Cashew Ranch Dressing (page 207).*

- *For some crunch, add 2 to 3 tablespoons soaked sunflower seeds to the burger mixture.*

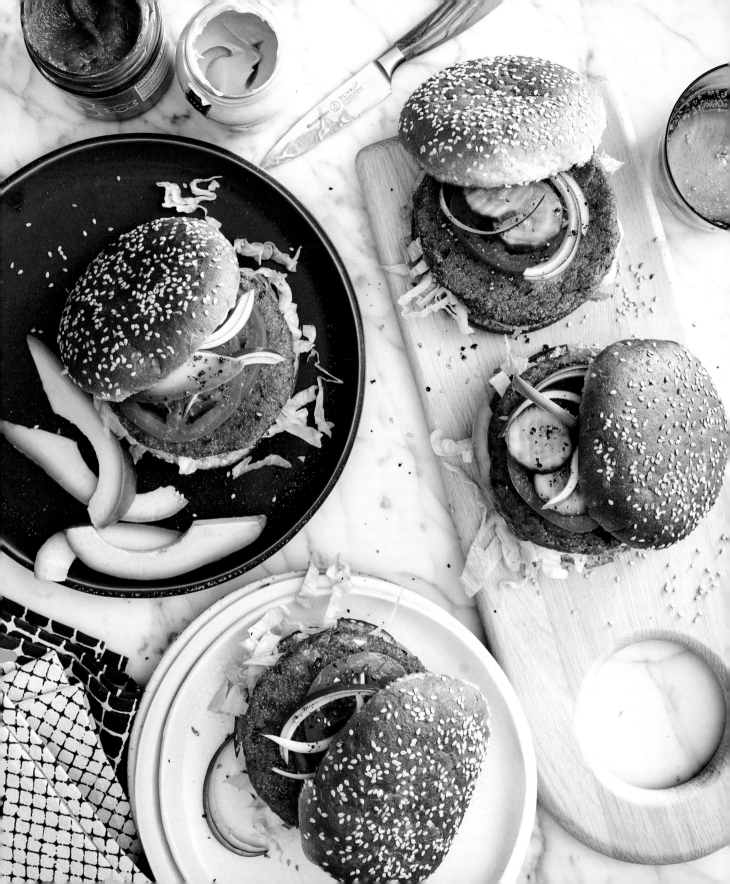

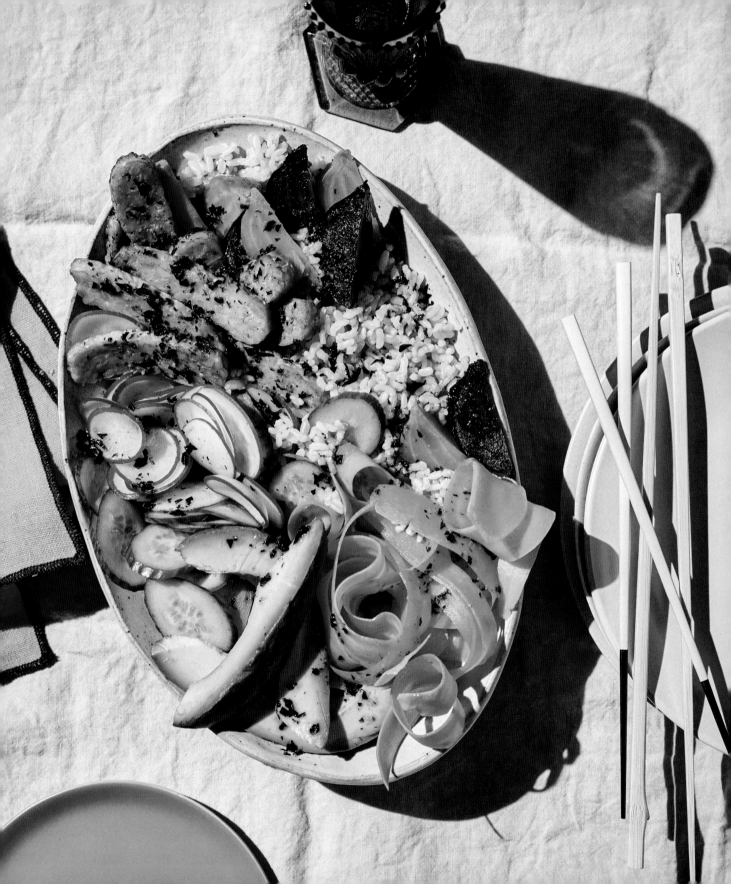

SUSHI TEMPEH BOWL
WITH TAMARI-GINGER DRESSING

FOR THE DRESSING

2 teaspoons EVOO

3 tablespoons reduced-sodium tamari or soy sauce

3 tablespoons rice wine vinegar

3 toasted nori sheets, finely chopped

Juice of 1 large orange or tangerine

3 teaspoons finely grated ginger

Dash of hot sauce

Freshly ground black pepper

FOR THE BOWL

1 8-ounce package tempeh, sliced thinly

1½ cups cooked brown rice

½ cup sliced radishes

1 ripe avocado, sliced

2 large carrots, spiralized or cut into ribbons

½ English cucumber, sliced thinly or spiralized

2 small cooked beets, cut into wedges

3 tablespoons toasted sesame seeds

NEURO 9 ITEMS: brown rice, tempeh, sesame seeds

PREP TIME: 15 minutes

COOKING TIME: 6 minutes

TOTAL TIME: 21 minutes

YIELD: 3 servings

Turn on the oven broiler. Whisk all dressing ingredients until well-combined; adjust the seasoning and set aside.

Brush the tempeh with half of the dressing and let marinate while you prepare your vegetables.

Arrange tempeh in a single layer on a baking sheet and generously brush with some dressing on both sides. Broil for about 3 minutes per side, flipping once and brushing with extra dressing. Alternatively, cook the tempeh on high heat in a nonstick pan for 3 minutes per side. Transfer to a plate and set aside.

Mix 2 to 3 tablespoons of the dressing into the rice and divide among three serving bowls. Arrange baked tempeh and the other ingredients on top, drizzle with the remaining dressing, and sprinkle with sesame seeds. Serve immediately.

Recipe Note

- *You can substitute the rice with riced vegetables, such as cauliflower, daikon radish, or jicama.*

SUPERFOOD PASTA
WITH HUMMUS WALNUT DRESSING

FOR THE DRESSING

⅔ cup oil-free hummus (see Recipe Notes, below)

6 tablespoons roughly chopped walnuts, divided

Zest and juice of 1 lemon (to taste)

Pinch of red pepper flakes

3 tablespoons fresh dill

Salt and freshly ground black pepper, to taste

FOR THE SALAD

2 cups thinly sliced lacinato kale, thick ribs removed

Juice of ½ lemon

½ box (4 ounces) whole-wheat penne pasta (or any other kind)

2 cups broccoli florets

⅔ cup frozen shelled edamame

1 medium carrot, peeled and grated

8 cherry tomatoes, halved

½ cup fresh blueberries

½ medium cucumber, thinly sliced

1 cup pea shoots or watercress

¼ cup fresh basil leaves, shredded

NEURO 9 ITEMS: hummus (chickpeas), broccoli, edamame, kale, blueberries, watercress, herbs and spices

PREP TIME: 15 minutes

COOKING TIME: 10–12 minutes

TOTAL TIME: 25–27 minutes

YIELD: 4 servings

Place the kale in a large bowl and add the lemon juice. Massage the kale for a minute to soften, then set aside. Boil the pasta according to package directions, adding the broccoli and edamame 2 to 3 minutes before the end of the cooking time. Drain in a colander, reserving 1 cup of the cooking liquid, and set aside to cool.

In a blender, blend the hummus, 3 tablespoons walnuts, lemon zest, and lemon juice until smooth, adding just enough of the cooled pasta cooking liquid to get a sauce consistency. Stir in red pepper flakes and dill. Season with salt and pepper to taste.

Place the cooled pasta, broccoli, and edamame into the large bowl with kale and toss with the dressing. Mix in the carrot, tomatoes, blueberries, cucumber, pea shoots or watercress, and basil.

Scatter the remaining 3 tablespoons walnuts on top and serve.

Recipe Notes

- *To make hummus, blend 2 cups drained cooked chickpeas with 2 garlic cloves, ¼ cup tahini, and the juice of 1 lemon in a blender until smooth, adding water as needed to get the desired consistency. Season with a dash of ground cumin, salt, and pepper and refrigerate for up to three days.*

- *You may substitute the whole-wheat penne pasta with brown rice or lentil pasta.*

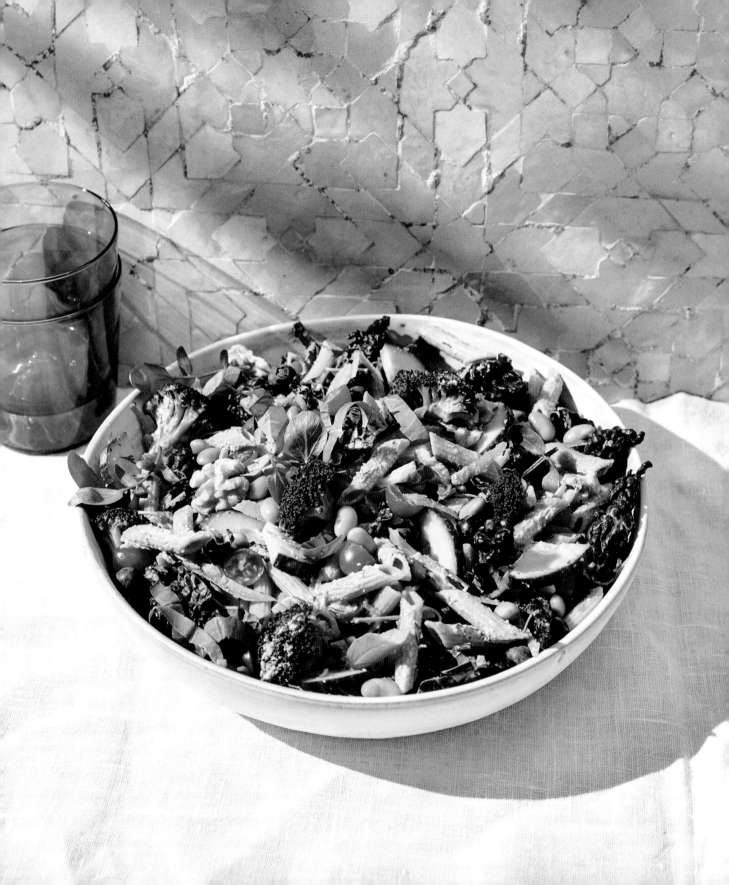

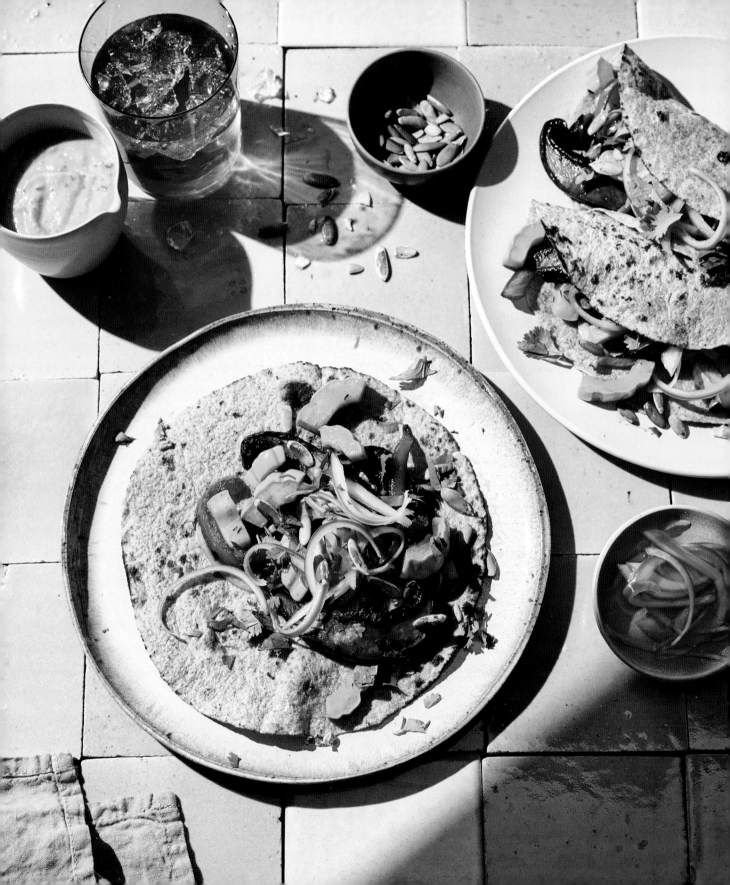

SPICY SQUASH AND PORTOBELLO TACOS

NEURO 9 ITEMS: pumpkin seeds, spices and herbs

PREP TIME: 20 minutes

COOKING TIME: 20–25 minutes

TOTAL TIME: 40–45 minutes

YIELD: 3 servings

Avocado oil spray

3 cups butternut, acorn, or delicata squash, seeded, peeled, and cubed

¼ teaspoon each of cayenne pepper and cumin (or to taste)

1 teaspoon dried thyme, divided

3 large portobello mushroom caps, sliced about ½-inch thick

1 medium red onion, sliced

2 garlic cloves, minced

1 chili in adobo sauce, minced

1½ tablespoons balsamic vinegar

1 teaspoon dried thyme

Salt and freshly ground black pepper, to taste

¼ cup pumpkin seeds or pine nuts, toasted

Handful of fresh parsley, chopped

100% whole wheat or sprouted whole wheat tortillas

Preheat the oven to 375°F; lightly spray two rimmed baking sheets with avocado oil cooking spray (or broth) or line with parchment paper. Set aside.

In a bowl, spray the squash with avocado oil then toss with cayenne pepper and cumin; season to taste with salt and pepper. Transfer to one of the prepared baking sheets and sprinkle with ½ teaspoon thyme.

Combine portobello caps, red onion slices, garlic, chili, and remaining thyme in a bowl; drizzle with the balsamic vinegar and season with salt and pepper to taste. Spread onto the other baking sheet. Spray with avocado oil or drizzle on some vegetable broth.

Place both sheets in the oven and bake, stirring occasionally, until the vegetables are cooked and begin to caramelize (about 15 to 20 minutes for the portobello mushrooms and 20 to 25 minutes for the squash). If needed, add a splash of water (or vegetable broth) to the baking sheets during the cooking process.

Toss the vegetables together, adjust seasoning if needed, and scatter pumpkin seeds and parsley on top. Use as a taco filling with sliced onions, guacamole, and salsa.

Recipe Note

- *Any leftovers can be used in salads or wraps, or serve with quinoa or your favorite whole grain.*

PLANTASTIC NEUROPLASTIC MEATBALLS

NEURO 9 ITEMS: quinoa, spinach, herbs and spices

PREP TIME: 20 minutes

COOKING TIME: 15 minutes

TOTAL TIME: 35 minutes

YIELD: 3 servings (3 to 4 meatballs per serving)

⅓ cup unsweetened plant-based milk of choice (or as needed)

1 slice 100% whole-wheat bread

1½ cups cooked quinoa

2 cups baby spinach, finely chopped

1 small beet, boiled and grated

1 medium sweet potato, boiled and mashed

½ cup cilantro leaves, chopped

1 teaspoon each of garlic powder, onion powder, paprika, and ground cumin

Juice and zest of 1 large lime

Sea salt and freshly ground black pepper, to taste

Oat flour or fresh 100% whole-wheat breadcrumbs (if needed)

EVOO spray for sautéing

Pour the milk over the bread slice and let soak for 5 minutes.

Preheat the oven to 400°F and line a baking sheet with parchment paper or a silicone baking mat.

Combine soaked bread, quinoa, spinach, beet, sweet potato, cilantro, garlic powder, onion powder, paprika, cumin, and lime zest and juice in a large mixing bowl. Season to taste and mix well, adjusting the consistency with a tablespoon of oat flour or breadcrumbs, if too soft.

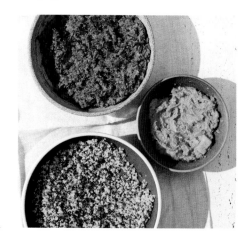

Using a 1½-inch scoop as a measure, form the mixture into balls. Place an oven-safe pan or iron skillet on medium heat, spray with EVOO, and sauté the meatballs so they are golden and crisp all around. Then arrange on the prepared baking sheet (or if you are using an iron skillet, keep them in the skillet) and bake for about 15 minutes or until golden. Let cool slightly and serve.

Recipe Notes

- *Add some spiciness to the mixture with a teaspoon of your favorite hot sauce.*

- *These are great on pasta with marinara sauce, in subs, or as is with Herbed Cauliflower Rice (page 165) and Spicy Green Hummus (page 206).*

- *You may form the mixture into burger patties and serve with a side of baked sweet potato fries and a crisp salad.*

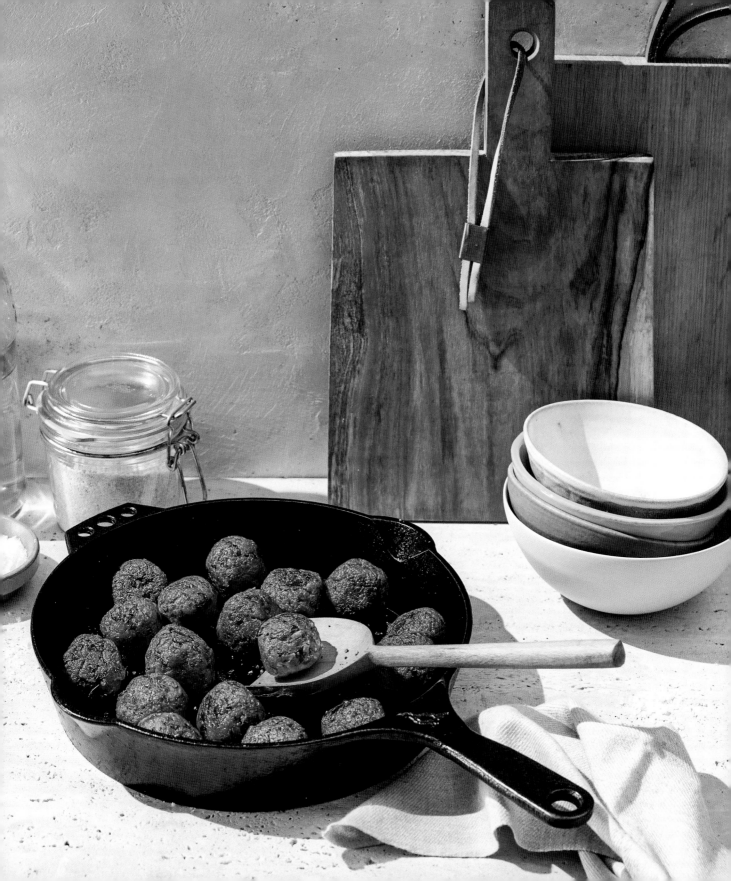

SPICY TOFU-GINGER QUINOA BOWL
WITH SHIITAKE MUSHROOMS

FOR THE DRESSING

1 4-ounce block silken tofu, drained

2 tablespoons tahini

2 teaspoons finely grated ginger (or to taste)

2 teaspoons sriracha or other hot chili sauce (or to taste)

½ cup fresh orange juice

1 tablespoon apple cider vinegar (or to taste)

Salt and freshly ground pepper, to taste

FOR THE BOWL

1 tablespoon EVOO

1 red chili pepper, thinly sliced

2 garlic cloves, minced

3 cups fresh mushrooms, sliced (any kind of mushroom)

1 tablespoon reduced-sodium tamari

1 cup frozen edamame, thawed

2 large carrots, cut into matchsticks or coarsely grated

2 cups sliced baby bok choy

1½ cups cooked quinoa

3 scallions, thinly sliced

¼ cup toasted peanuts or cashews, coarsely chopped

NEURO 9 ITEMS: tofu, tahini, quinoa, edamame, bok choy, nuts and spices

PREP TIME: 20 minutes

COOKING TIME: 10 minutes

TOTAL TIME: 30 minutes

YIELD: 3 servings

Whisk all dressing ingredients in a bowl, thinning with a little water, if needed, to get the desired consistency; season to taste and refrigerate until needed.

Heat 1 tablespoon EVOO in a wok or large nonstick skillet over medium-high heat. Add red chili and garlic; cook, stirring, for 10 seconds, then add the mushrooms, tamari, and edamame. Cook, stirring often, until tender (5 to 6 minutes), then add the carrots and bok choy and cook for about 1 minute. If too dry, add a splash of vegetable broth. Remove from the heat and set aside.

Toss the cooked quinoa with a few tablespoons of the dressing, adjust the seasoning, and divide among three serving bowls. Pile the stir-fried mixture over the quinoa and drizzle with the dressing. Scatter scallions and peanuts over the top and serve.

Recipe Note

• *You can use lima beans instead of edamame.*

RICED CAULI GRILLED TOFU BOWL

FOR THE TOFU

Juice of ½ lemon

1 garlic clove, minced

2 teaspoons tamari

1½ tablespoons nutritional yeast

1 teaspoon dried oregano

1 12-ounce block extra-firm tofu, drained, pressed in a towel for at least 20 minutes, and sliced into 4 thick slices

Salt and freshly ground black pepper, to taste

FOR THE BOWL

EVOO spray

3 scallions, chopped

1 garlic clove, minced

4 cups riced cauliflower

1 cup grated carrots

3 tablespoons dukkah spice mix, divided (or to taste)

Handful each of fresh flat-leaf parsley and mint, roughly chopped

Salt and freshly ground pepper, to taste

1 cup cooked edamame or broad beans, drained

¼ cup pitted green olives

½ cup cherry tomatoes, halved

1 cup sliced cucumbers, sliced

NEURO 9 ITEMS: tofu, cauliflower, edamame or broad beans, herbs and spices

PREP TIME: 10 minutes

COOKING TIME: 10 minutes

TOTAL TIME: 20 minutes plus 30 minutes for marinating

YIELD: 3 servings

Mix lemon juice, garlic, tamari, nutritional yeast, and oregano and rub tofu slices with the mixture. Season with salt and pepper and set aside to marinate for 30 minutes.

Heat a large skillet over medium heat and add EVOO, scallions, garlic, cauliflower rice, and carrot. Cook, stirring occasionally, for 4 to 5 minutes, until the cauliflower is just tender, adding a tablespoon of water if needed. Turn off the heat and gently stir in 2 tablespoons dukkah, and the parsley and mint. Season to taste and set aside.

Heat a grill pan, spray lightly with EVOO, and grill the tofu slices, carefully flipping once, for about 2 to 3 minutes per side or until grill marks appear. Alternatively, broil the tofu in the oven.

Divide the cauliflower rice among three serving bowls and top with the tofu, edamame, olives, tomatoes, and cucumbers. Sprinkle with the remaining dukkah and serve.

Recipe Notes

- *To make cauliflower rice, see instructions in the Herbed Cauliflower Rice (page 165).*

- *Replace dukkah with sesame seeds, cumin, and coriander.*

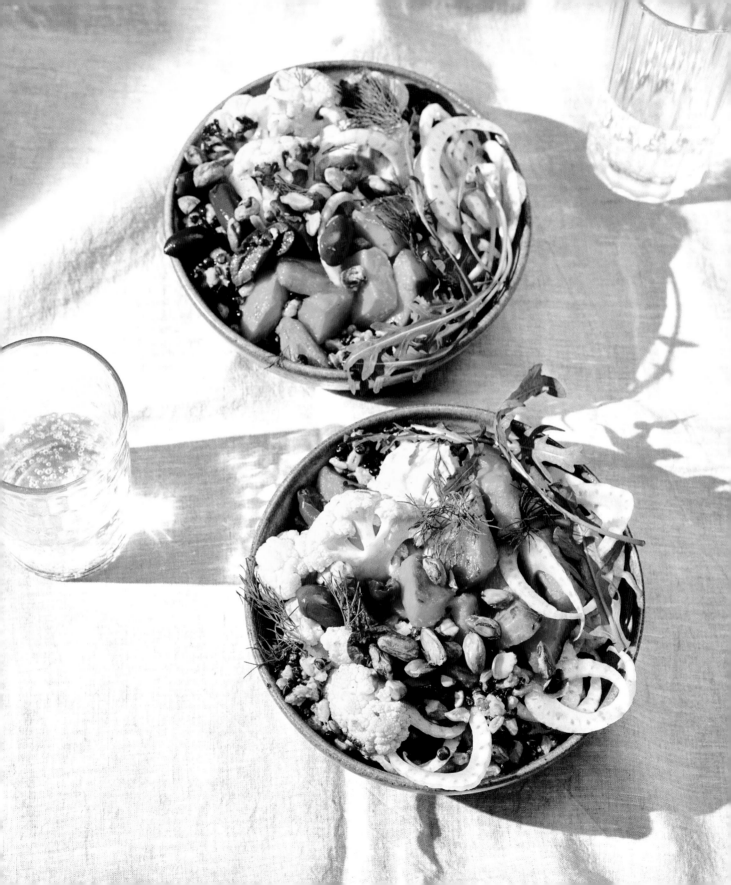

MEDITERRANEAN LONGEVITY BOWL

FOR THE DRESSING

1 garlic clove, minced

3 tablespoons tahini

2 tablespoons white balsamic vinegar (or apple cider vinegar)

Juice of 1 lemon

½ teaspoon harissa and/or whole-grain Dijon mustard (optional)

1 teaspoon za'atar (or substitute dried thyme or oregano) plus more for serving

Sea salt and freshly ground black pepper, to taste

FOR THE BOWL

1½ cups cooked Puy or beluga lentils

1 cup cooked farro

6 tablespoons hummus

2 cups roasted mixed vegetables (recipe on page 175)

1 fennel bulb, thinly sliced

2 large handfuls of arugula (or any other tender greens)

¼ cup pitted Kalamata olives

¼ cup lightly toasted pistachios, roughly chopped

NEURO 9 ITEMS: lentils, farro, hummus, arugula, pistachios, tahini, herbs and spices

PREP TIME: 10 minutes

COOKING TIME: none

TOTAL TIME: 10 minutes

YIELD: 3 servings

Whisk together all dressing ingredients until smooth and creamy, adding enough water to obtain a pourable dressing consistency. Season to taste with salt and pepper.

In a large bowl, combine lentils and farro and toss with half of the dressing. Divide the mixture among three serving bowls and add 2 tablespoons hummus on one side of each bowl. Arrange roasted vegetables, fennel, arugula, and olives around the hummus. Drizzle the vegetables with the remaining dressing and sprinkle with pistachios and extra za'atar before serving.

GREEK GIGANTES

1 tablespoon EVOO

½ onion, sliced into moon-shaped slivers the size of the broad beans

2 garlic cloves, minced

1 15-ounce can no salt added diced tomatoes with juice

1 tablespoon tomato paste

1 teaspoon turmeric

½ teaspoon black pepper

1 teaspoon oregano

1 teaspoon fresh or dried thyme

1 15-ounce can giant or butter beans, or 10-ounce package dried beans, cooked

2 cups finely chopped greens (such as spinach, Swiss chard, or lacinato kale)

½ small serrano pepper, deseeded and finely chopped (for heat, optional)

Salt, to taste

½ cup chopped parsley, for garnish

NEURO 9 ITEMS: giant beans, greens, 100% whole-wheat bread, spices (including herbs and turmeric)

PREP TIME: 15 minutes (if the giant beans are cooked)

COOKING TIME: 35 minutes

TOTAL TIME: 50 minutes

YIELD: 2 servings

Heat a Dutch oven or heavy deep pan on high heat. Add the EVOO and onions; cook for 2 minutes. Add the garlic and cook for another minute. Add the chopped tomatoes, tomato paste, and spices and cook for 10 minutes. Then add the beans; cover with a lid. Lower heat to medium-low and cook for about 20 minutes until the flavors mix and the color deepens.

During the last 5 minutes of cooking, stir in greens and serrano pepper for heat (optional). Add salt to taste. Serve in a deep bowl with chopped parsley as garnish.

Serve with a slice of crusty 100% whole-wheat sourdough bread or brown rice.

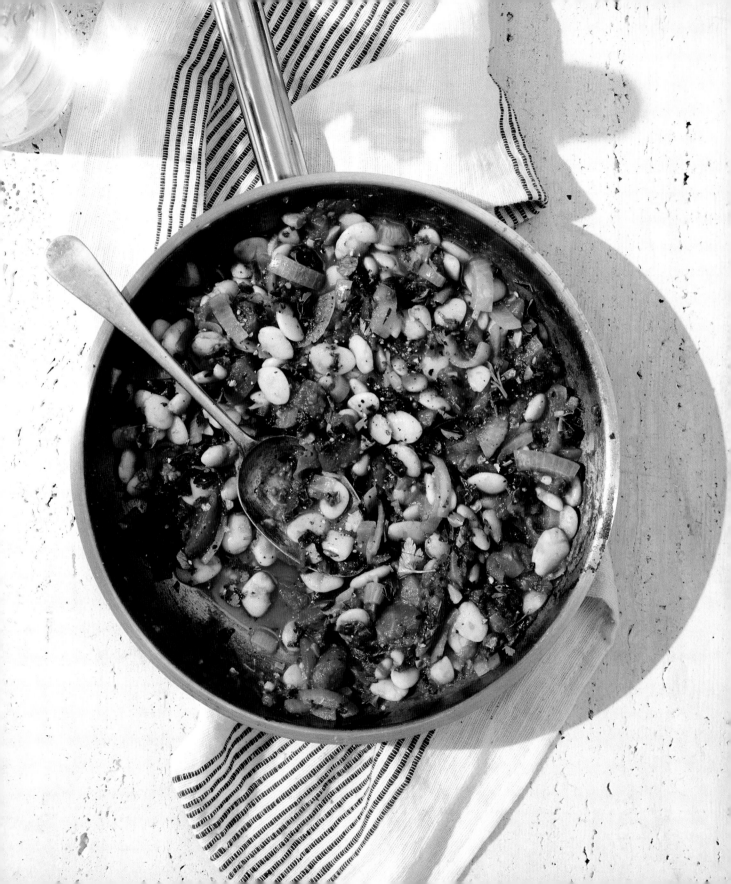

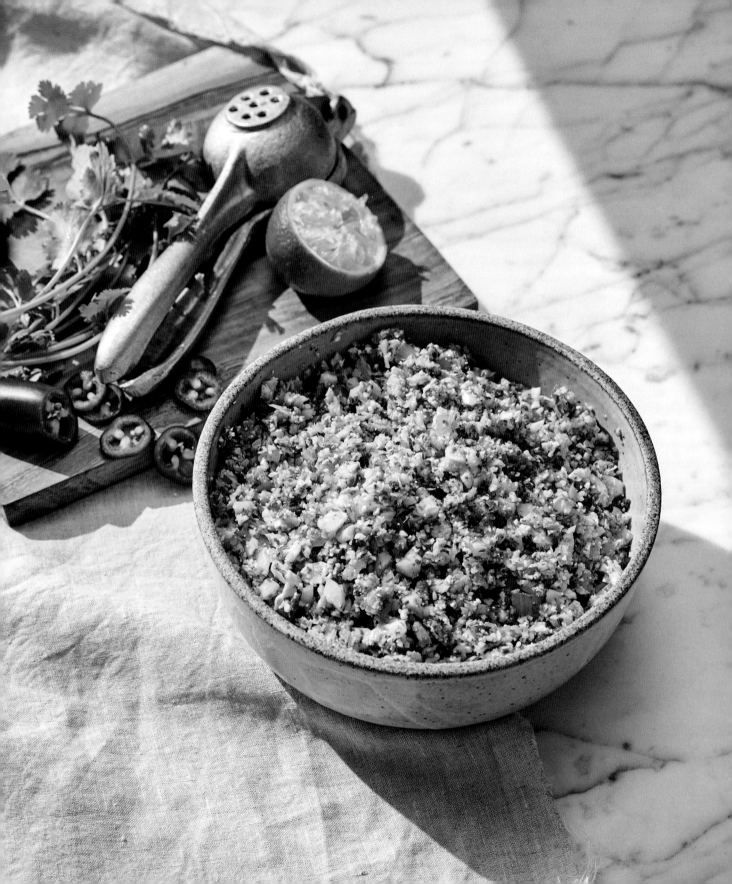

HERBED CAULIFLOWER RICE

NEURO 9 ITEMS: cauliflower, herbs

PREP TIME: 10 minutes

COOKING TIME: 10 minutes

TOTAL TIME: 20 minutes

YIELD: 4 servings

1 large head cauliflower, riced (about 4 cups), or 1-pound bag cauliflower rice

1 medium jalapeño pepper, seeds and pith removed, chopped

2 cups cilantro leaves, large stems removed, chopped (or substitute parsley or dill)

2 tablespoons lime juice

1 tablespoon EVOO

½ cup chopped white or yellow onion

2 garlic cloves, minced

Salt and pepper to taste

Remove the leaves and stems from the cauliflower and cut the cauliflower into four quarters. If you're using a box grater, use the medium grating side and grate the cauliflower into "rice." If you're using a food processor, use the grater blade, cut the cauliflower into smaller pieces, and feed into the food processor and grate. Set aside.

Place the jalapeño pepper, cilantro, salt, and lime juice in the food processor using an "S" blade, and process until a loose paste is formed. Set aside.

Heat a large saucepan, Dutch oven, or skillet (with a lid) over medium heat. Once hot, spray with EVOO and add the onion, garlic, and a pinch of salt and sauté 2 to 3 minutes, stirring occasionally. Then add the cauliflower rice. Stir to cook for 2 minutes. Cover and steam for 1 to 2 minutes. Remove from heat. Be careful not to make it too soft and mushy.

Add the cilantro mixture and stir to coat. Cook for 1 more minute on medium heat, stirring frequently.

Remove from heat. Taste and adjust flavor with salt or lime juice as needed. Serve with fresh cilantro and lime if desired.

Cauliflower rice is best when fresh, but it will keep in the refrigerator up to two days.

TACO QUINOA

NEURO 9 ITEMS: quinoa, spices

PREP TIME: 15 minutes

COOKING TIME: 55–60 minutes

TOTAL TIME: 70–75 minutes

YIELD: 6 servings

1 cup tricolor or red quinoa, rinsed thoroughly with water

1¾ cups low-sodium vegetable broth

½ cup salsa

2 tablespoons nutritional yeast

2 teaspoons ground cumin

2 teaspoons ground chili powder

1 teaspoon garlic powder

Salt and freshly ground pepper, to taste

EVOO spray

Heat a medium saucepan over medium heat. Once hot, add rinsed quinoa and toast 4 to 5 minutes, stirring frequently.

Add vegetable broth and bring to a boil over medium-high heat. Reduce heat to low, cover with a lid, and cook 20 to 25 minutes, or until liquid is completely absorbed. Remove from heat, fluff quinoa with a fork, and let rest for 10 minutes partially covered.

Preheat the oven to 375°F. In a large bowl, mix the cooked quinoa with the remaining ingredients—salsa, nutritional yeast, cumin, chili powder, garlic powder, salt, and pepper. Toss to combine.

Line a baking sheet with parchment paper and spread the quinoa mixture on the baking sheet. Spray with EVOO and bake for 30 minutes, stirring/tossing once after 15 minutes to ensure even baking. When the quinoa is toasty and brown, remove from the oven.

Serve as is with baked corn chips, salsa, and guacamole; or as filling in tacos, burritos, enchiladas, and peppers; or as a topping in soups and salads.

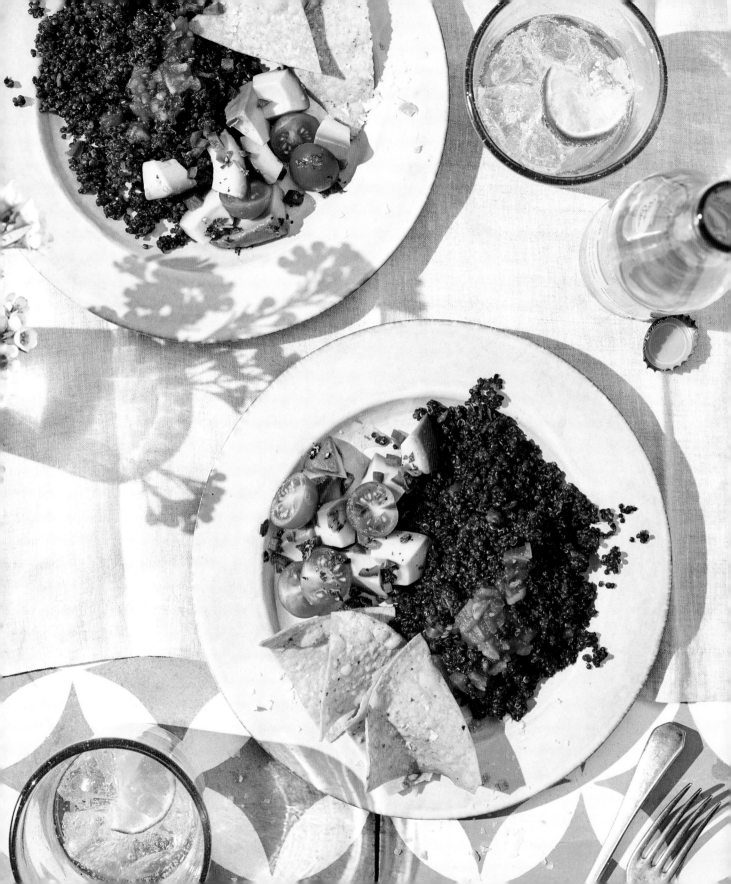

BRAINY TABOULEH

FOR THE SALAD

½ cup bulgur wheat, cooked according to package instructions and cooled

1½ tablespoons hemp seeds

⅓ cup each of fresh mint, fresh Italian parsley, and baby arugula, chopped

⅓ cup pomegranate seeds

3 scallions, chopped

1 large cucumber, peeled, seeded, and diced

2 medium tomatoes, seeded and diced

FOR THE DRESSING

½ ripe avocado, diced

2 tablespoons tahini

Juice of 1 lemon

1 garlic clove, crushed

Salt and freshly ground black pepper, to taste

NEURO 9 ITEMS: bulgur wheat, hemp seeds, pomegranate seeds, scallions, tahini, herbs and spices

PREP TIME: 20 minutes

COOKING TIME: none

TOTAL TIME: 20 minutes

YIELD: 3 servings

Prepare all salad ingredients in a mixing bowl and toss lightly to combine.

In a blender, blend together all dressing ingredients, adding just enough water to get a smooth and creamy dressing consistency. Season with salt and pepper to taste. Drizzle dressing on the salad ingredients and toss thoroughly.

Recipe Notes

- *Substitute bulgur with whole-wheat couscous, quinoa, or riced cauliflower.*

- *Sprinkle on some sumac for even more flavor.*

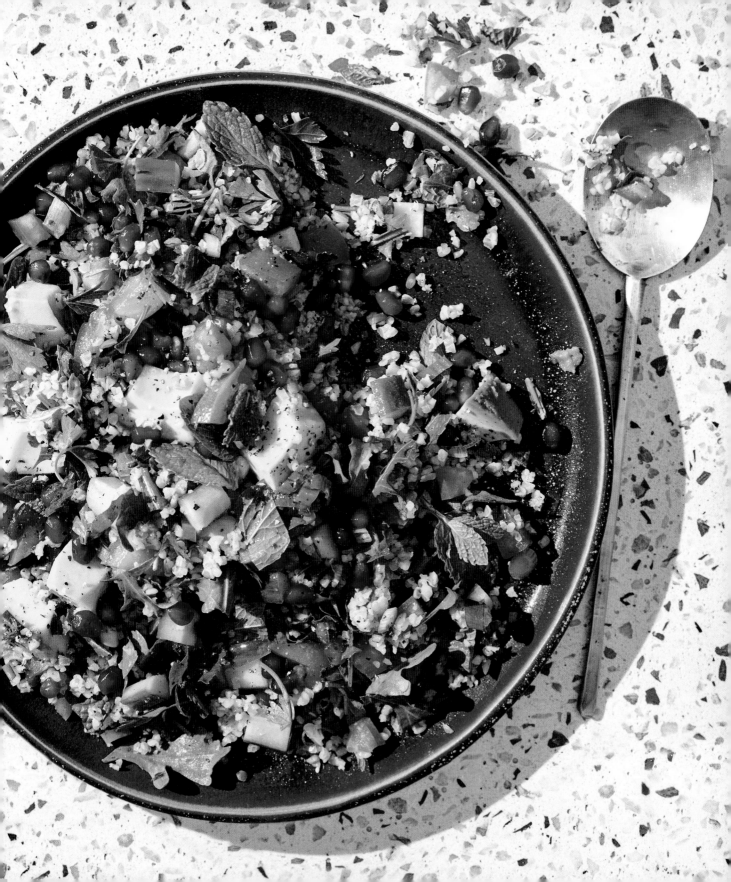

ROASTED ROOT VEGETABLES

Nutrient-dense and low in calories, root vegetables are packed with antioxidants, fiber, vitamins, and minerals and provide many health benefits—from regulating blood sugar to feeding gut bacteria, which in turn produce chemicals that boost brain function.

There are many varieties of root vegetables, from the popular sweet potatoes, yams, beets, carrots, onions, ginger, and garlic to the less familiar celeriac, jicama, Jerusalem artichokes, rutabagas, and turnips. They all deserve attention because of their individual nutritional profiles. Easily available year-round, root vegetables are quite versatile and can be boiled, baked, mashed, or roasted; some, like carrots, beets, and jicama, can be eaten raw.

Roasting brings out the vegetables' sweetness and mellows their earthy flavor. The roasting techniques are a bit different if you decide to cook with oil or without oil. Oil acts as a "sealant," keeping the moisture trapped inside the vegetables such that the inside gets soft and the outside gets crispy.

FOR COOKING WITH OIL: Select firm vegetables, peel, and cut them to the same size to ensure even cooking. Toss with 1 to 2 tablespoons avocado oil in a large bowl before you place them in the pan. Don't drizzle oil in the pan. Most of the oil won't coat the vegetables that way and will be wasted. If you are using an oil spray, you can spray directly on the vegetables in the pan.

Keep seasoning simple: salt, pepper, a few minced garlic cloves, fresh or dried thyme or rosemary.

Use a metal baking sheet or a shallow roasting pan. Don't use a glass pan.

Don't crowd the roasting pan. Spread the vegetables in one layer. If you pile them, they will steam, not roast.

Preheat the oven to 375°F. High heat will roast the veggies and preserve moisture inside.

Roast the vegetables for about 35 to 45 minutes or until golden and slightly caramelized. Flip halfway for uniform cooking.

Veggies will keep refrigerated in an airtight container for up to three days.

FOR OIL-FREE ROASTING: Steam or quickly boil the root vegetables first. For boiling, fill a large stockpot a third full with water and bring to a boil. Peel the vegetables and cut them to relatively equal sizes. Put the cut vegetables in the pot and add additional water until the vegetables are covered. Boil for 7 minutes until they are tender—a knife should easily pierce them. Remove from water with a perforated spoon and place on a roasting pan or a baking sheet with herbs and spices to roast.

For steaming, fill a skillet with water, bring to a boil, and carefully place a colander or steamer basket over the water, not immersed. Place peeled and cut vegetables in the steamer and cover with a lid. Steam for about 7 minutes until tender. Then place them in a roasting pan or a baking sheet with herbs and spices to roast.

Use the following recipe (with oil) as a guide and tailor it to your taste with any root vegetables you have on hand. Serve the roasted vegetables as a hearty and nourishing side, or add to soups, pasta, rice dishes, or salads.

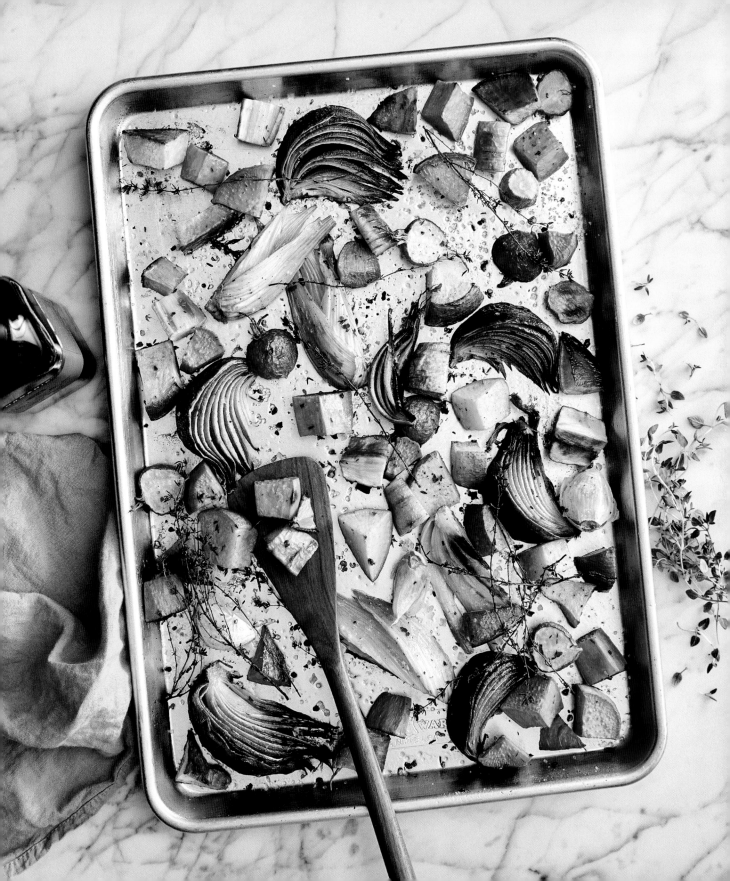

PREP TIME: 10 minutes

COOKING TIME: 30–40 minutes

TOTAL TIME: 40–50 minutes

YIELD: 3 servings

1 pound mixed root vegetables, peeled and cut into equal-size chunks

1 red onion, quartered

1 small fennel bulb, quartered

4 garlic cloves, whole and unpeeled

Salt and freshly ground pepper, to taste

½ teaspoon red pepper flakes

1 tablespoon avocado oil

2 sprigs of fresh rosemary or thyme, chopped

Preheat the oven to 375°F. Line a metal baking sheet or shallow roasting pan with parchment paper or a silicone baking mat.

Combine root vegetables, onion, fennel, and garlic cloves in a large bowl and season to taste with salt, pepper, and pepper flakes. Add the avocado oil or spray, if using, and toss to coat.

Transfer to the prepared baking sheet, spreading in a single layer, and add the rosemary. Do not crowd the vegetables.

Roast, stirring occasionally, for 30 to 40 minutes, or until the vegetables are cooked through and begin to caramelize. Discard the garlic cloves and rosemary sprigs. It's best to serve the veggies warm, but they can be served cold as well. Store them in a glass, airtight container in the refrigerator and use within four or five days.

Recipe Note

- *Use avocado oil instead of EVOO during baking for its high smoke point.*

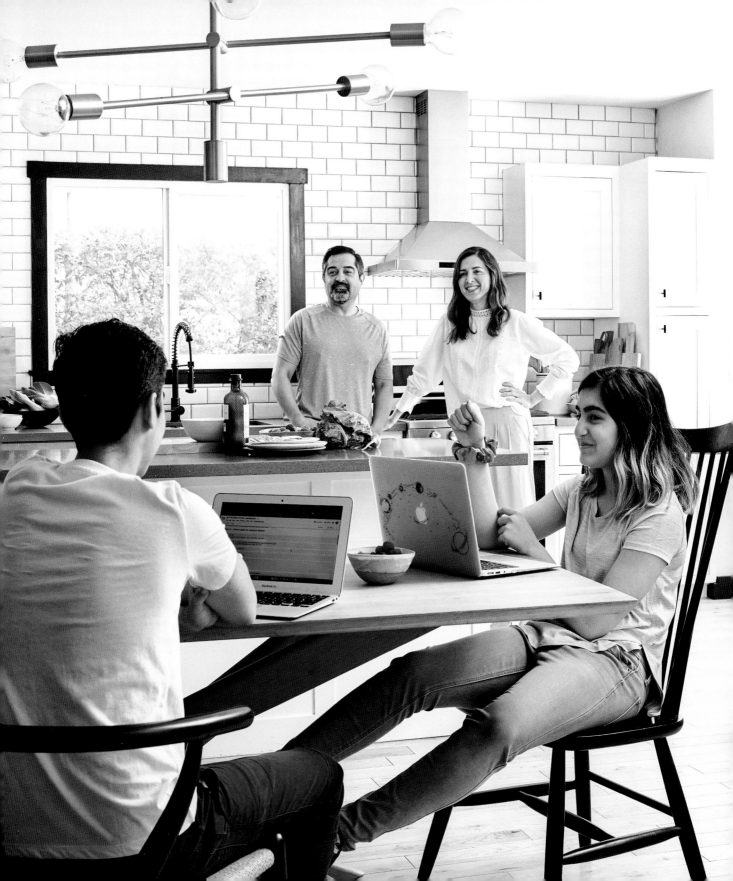

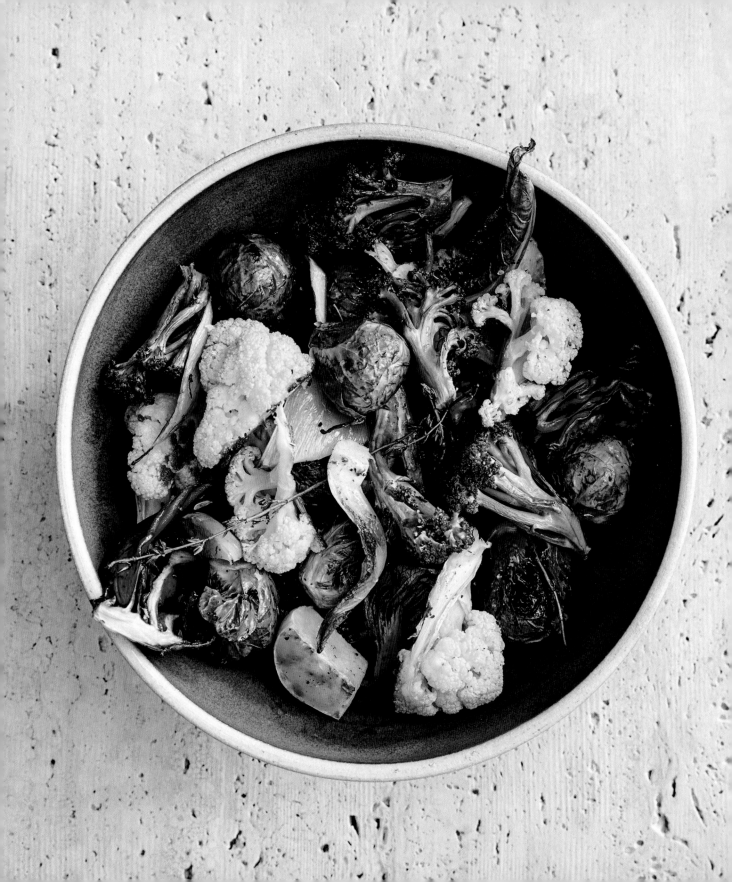

ROASTED CRUCIFEROUS VEGETABLES

1½ cups Brussels sprouts, halved

2 cups cauliflower florets, cut into bite-size pieces

1 cup kohlrabi, peeled and cut into bite-size pieces

2 cups broccoli florets, cut into bite-size pieces

2 cups roughly chopped cabbage

2 cups trimmed and roughly chopped bok choy

2 garlic cloves, minced

1 teaspoon mixed dried herbs or Italian seasoning (or any spice mix, such as curry powder)

¼ teaspoon cayenne pepper or mustard powder

Salt and freshly ground black pepper, to taste

3 tablespoons balsamic vinegar

1 to 2 tablespoons avocado oil or avocado oil spray

⅓ cup low-sodium vegetable broth (more as needed)

PREP TIME: 10–15 minutes

COOKING TIME: 20–25 minutes

TOTAL TIME: 30–40 minutes

YIELD: 3 servings

Preheat the oven to 400°F and line a large rimmed baking sheet with parchment paper or a silicone baking mat.

Combine Brussels sprouts, cauliflower, kohlrabi, broccoli, cabbage, bok choy, garlic, herbs, and cayenne pepper in a large bowl and season to taste with salt and pepper. Drizzle with balsamic vinegar and avocado oil, if using, and add vegetable broth; toss until evenly coated.

Spread the vegetables onto the prepared baking sheet and roast, stirring occasionally, for about 20 to 25 minutes, or until cooked to your taste and slightly caramelized. If necessary, add a splash of vegetable broth during roasting.

Recipe Note

- *Fresh vegetables roast best, but if using frozen ones, set the oven temperature to 425°F and roast for 25 minutes.*

CORTICAL CAULIFLOWER WITH WALNUT SAUCE

1 teaspoon smoked paprika

2 tablespoons Italian or herbes de Provence seasoning blend (or 1 tablespoon each of thyme and rosemary mixed with ½ tablespoon each of basil and sage)

1 head cauliflower, cut into 3 (1-inch-thick) slices

1 tablespoon avocado oil or avocado oil spray

Salt and freshly ground pepper, to taste

OPTIONAL GARNISHES

Chopped fresh parsley, pepper flakes, toasted pine nuts, and capers

FOR THE SAUCE

1 cup toasted walnuts

2 garlic cloves, minced

¼ cup tahini

Zest and juice of 1 large lemon

2 teaspoons liquid aminos, or low-sodium tamari or soy sauce

2 tablespoons nutritional yeast

Freshly ground black pepper

NEURO 9 ITEMS: cauliflower, walnuts, herbs and spices

PREP TIME: 20 minutes

COOKING TIME: 20 minutes

TOTAL TIME: 40 minutes

YIELD: 3 servings

Preheat the oven to 425°F and line a rimmed baking sheet with parchment paper or a silicone baking mat.

Mix paprika and Italian seasoning; lightly brush the cauliflower steaks with avocado oil and rub with the paprika mixture. Season to taste with salt and freshly ground pepper.

Arrange the steaks on the prepared baking sheet and roast, flipping halfway through, until tender and golden brown, about 15 to 20 minutes.

In a blender, blend all sauce ingredients, adding enough water to get the desired consistency; season to taste, and set aside.

Place a slice on a plate, cover with sauce, and top with desired garnishes. Serve with a side salad.

Recipe Note

- *After cutting the cauliflower, reserve any leftover cauliflower for another use or roast pieces alongside the slices and refrigerate for up to five days (add to salads and soups).*

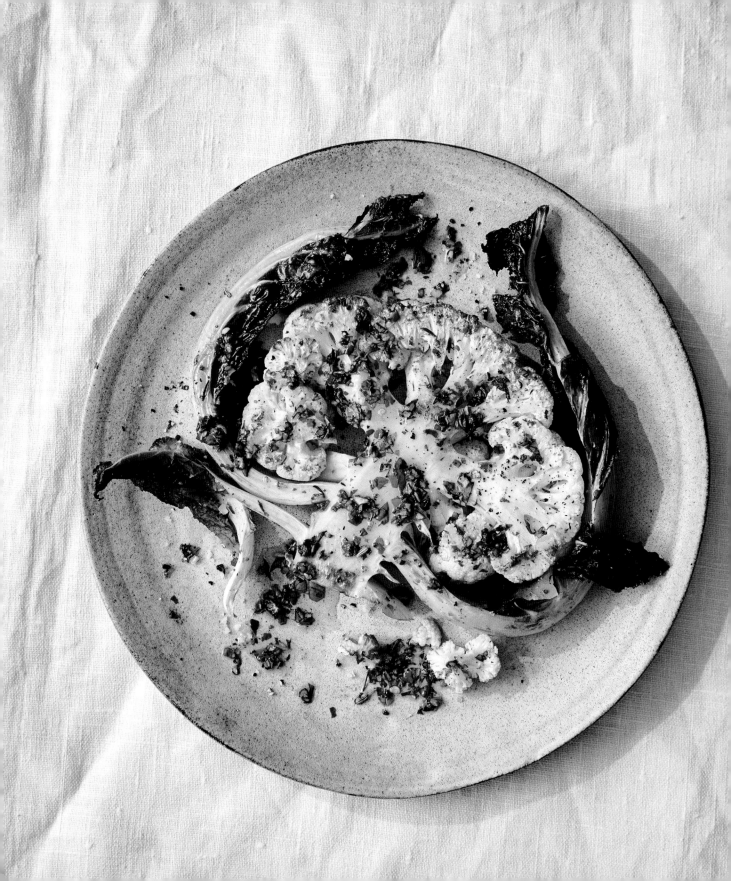

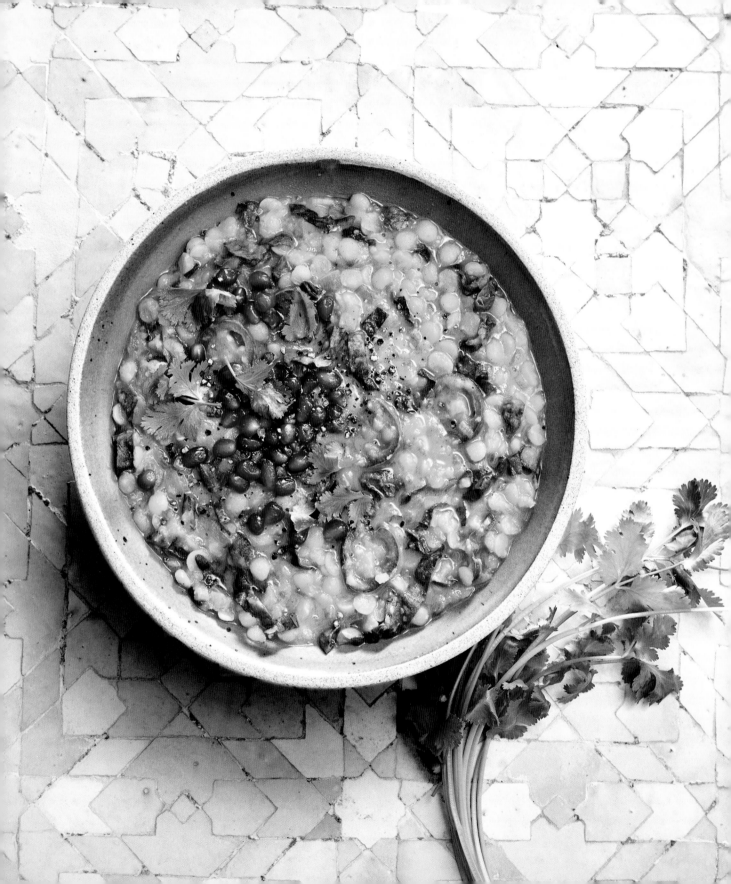

YELLOW SPLIT PEA SOUP WITH SPINACH AND POMEGRANATE

1½ cups yellow split peas, rinsed

2 medium tomatoes, peeled, deseeded, and diced small

5 cups low-sodium vegetable broth

½ tablespoon EVOO

1 medium onion, finely chopped

1 hot green chili, thinly sliced

1 teaspoon finely grated fresh ginger

2 garlic cloves, minced

1 teaspoon each of ground cumin, garam masala, and ground turmeric

3 cups spinach

½ tablespoon apple cider vinegar (or to taste)

Salt and freshly ground black pepper, to taste

3 tablespoons pomegranate seeds

2 tablespoons cilantro leaves

NEURO 9 ITEMS: yellow split peas, spinach, spices

PREP TIME: 10 minutes

COOKING TIME: 40 minutes

TOTAL TIME: 50 minutes

YIELD: 4 servings

Rinse the split peas and put in a large pot with tomatoes and vegetable broth; bring to a boil. Reduce the heat to low, cover partially, and simmer, skimming the foam occasionally, until the split peas are tender, about 30 minutes. You may need to add a little water during the process if it thickens too much.

Heat a large skillet over medium heat, add EVOO and onion and sauté until translucent, about 4 minutes. Add the green chili, ginger, and garlic and cook, stirring often, for about 1 minute, then add the cumin, garam masala, and turmeric. Add a tablespoon of broth as you cook to deglaze the skillet. Stir in a ladle of the split peas and then tip the mixture into the pot, stirring to incorporate.

Bring the soup to a boil, then add the spinach and season to taste; cook for about 5 minutes, until the spinach has wilted. If desired, blend with an immersion blender.

Adjust seasoning if needed, ladle the soup into bowls, and scatter pomegranate seeds and cilantro on top before serving.

CHICKPEA BARLEY SOUP

½ tablespoon EVOO

1 leek, thinly sliced

1 celery stalk, chopped

1 medium carrot, diced small

1 cup mushrooms, roughly chopped

1 cup uncooked hulled barley (or pearled barley for shorter cooking time)

5 cups low-sodium vegetable broth

1 large bunch of collard greens or beet tops (leaves only), thinly sliced

1 15.5-ounce can chickpeas, drained and rinsed

Salt and freshly ground black pepper, to taste

2 tablespoons each of chopped fresh dill and chives

Juice of 1 large lemon

NEURO 9 ITEMS: collard greens or beet tops, chickpeas, herbs and spices
PREP TIME: 10 minutes
COOKING TIME: 50–70 minutes
TOTAL TIME: 60–80 minutes
YIELD: 4 servings

Heat the EVOO in a large saucepan and add the leek, celery, carrot, and mushrooms. Cook over medium heat, stirring occasionally, for about 5 minutes, or until tender.

Add the barley and stir for a couple of minutes, then pour in the broth. Bring to a boil and lower the heat to medium-low; simmer for about 50 minutes or until barley is tender. If you are using pearled barley, cook for 30 minutes.

Once the barley is softened, add collard greens and chickpeas, season to taste, and continue cooking for 5 to 10 minutes or until the collard greens have wilted.

Stir in dill, chives, and lemon juice and serve.

Recipe Note

- *Serve the soup with a dollop of Cashew Sour Cream (page 205) mixed with a dash of hot sauce.*

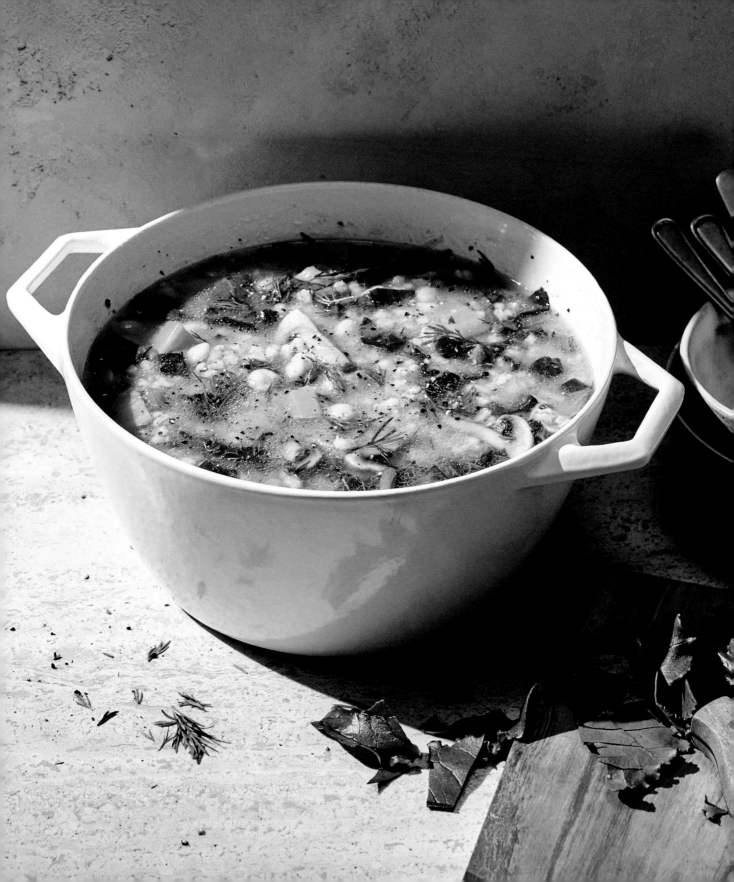

HEARTY BEAN CHILI

1 teaspoon EVOO

1 large onion, finely chopped

1 large green or red bell pepper, diced (to the size of beans)

1 large jalapeño, seeds and pith removed, finely chopped

½ teaspoon salt

6 garlic cloves, minced

2 tablespoons ground cumin

1 tablespoon dried oregano

3 tablespoons chili powder

1 teaspoon smoked paprika

½ teaspoon black pepper

2 15-ounce cans no salt added crushed tomatoes

3 tablespoons tomato paste

3 cups water, divided, plus more as needed

1 15-ounce can pinto beans, drained

1 15-ounce can black beans, drained

1 15-ounce can kidney beans, drained

Salt and freshly ground pepper, to taste

Juice of 2 limes

OPTIONAL GARNISHES
Avocado slices, chopped red onion, chopped cilantro, chopped jalapeño, and Cashew Sour Cream (page 205)

NEURO 9 ITEMS: beans, herbs and spices

PREP TIME: 10 minutes

COOKING TIME: 45 minutes

TOTAL TIME: 55 minutes

YIELD: 6 servings

Heat a 4-quart pot over medium heat. Add EVOO and onion and cook for 2 minutes. Add bell pepper and jalapeño. Cook for 3 minutes until the peppers are soft and fragrant. Add garlic and sauté for 30 seconds. Add cumin, oregano, chili powder, paprika, salt, and pepper and stir to make the spices more fragrant and toasty for about 1 minute. Add the crushed tomatoes and tomato paste and cook for about 3 minutes.

Then add 2 cups of the water to deglaze.

Add the beans and stir. Add the additional cup of water if needed. The beans should be submerged in the liquid and not look too dry. Cover the pot, lower the heat, and simmer for about 30 minutes. Add more water if the chili cooks down too much.

After 30 minutes, turn off the heat. Adjust the taste with salt or pepper as needed. Add the lime juice. For more heat, add more sliced jalapeños.

Serve in bowls with garnishes of your choice. This chili is great with Cornbread Muffins (page 217).

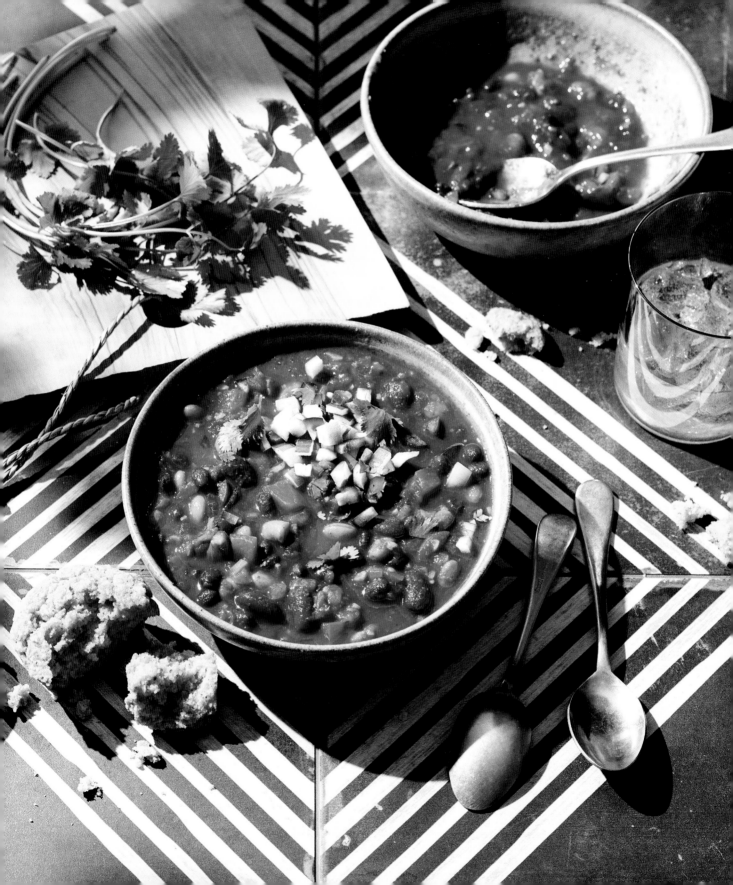

KALE BUTTERNUT SQUASH AND SPICED CHICKPEA SALAD

NEURO 9 ITEMS: chickpeas, spices (including turmeric), kale

PREP TIME: 20 minutes

COOKING TIME: 25 minutes

TOTAL TIME: 45 minutes

YIELD: 6 servings

FOR THE SALAD

1 1-pound butternut squash, peeled, cored, and cut into 1-inch pieces

EVOO spray

1 15-ounce can no salt added chickpeas, rinsed and drained

Pinch of salt

½ teaspoon black pepper

½ teaspoon turmeric

½ teaspoon smoked paprika

½ teaspoon garlic powder

½ teaspoon cayenne pepper (optional)

2 bundles kale, destemmed and roughly chopped

1 tablespoon fresh lemon juice

FOR THE DRESSING

⅓ cup tahini

1 garlic clove, minced

3 tablespoons lemon juice

1 tablespoon monk fruit sweetener

Pinch of salt

Water to thin (about ½ cup)

Preheat the oven to 400°F. Line a large baking sheet with parchment paper or a silicone baking mat and spread the squash out in a single layer. Do not crowd, so the pieces will cook uniformly and not steam. Spray with EVOO and sprinkle with a pinch of salt; place in oven. Flip pieces after about 15 minutes. Let cook for 25 minutes total. Squash is done when the edges are browned slightly on the outside and it's fork-tender on the inside. Remove from the oven and allow to cool.

Prepare the chickpeas while the squash is baking. Drain chickpeas and remove any loose skin. Heat a nonstick pan on high heat. Place the chickpeas in the pan and spray with some EVOO. Sauté, stirring the chickpeas or shaking the pan to roll the chickpeas for even cooking. Add the spices after 3 minutes and roll the chickpeas until the outsides are dry and crisped, for a total of 10 minutes. Remove from heat and set aside.

Place the kale into a large mixing bowl and sprinkle with lemon juice. Massage for about 3 minutes.

Whisk tahini, garlic, lemon juice, monk fruit sweetener, and salt in a medium mixing bowl. Slowly add the water until creamy and pourable. The mixture may seize up and thicken at first, but continue adding water a little at a time, whisking until desired consistency. Taste and adjust flavor as needed, adding more lemon juice for acidity, or salt to taste.

Add half of the dressing to the kale and toss. Add the squash and half of the chickpeas and toss gently. Sprinkle the rest of the chickpeas and drizzle the rest of the dressing on top as needed. Serve immediately.

Recipe Note

- *You can use sweet potatoes instead of butternut squash. If you don't have time to cook the squash or potatoes, use one or two diced sweet apples, such as gala apples.*

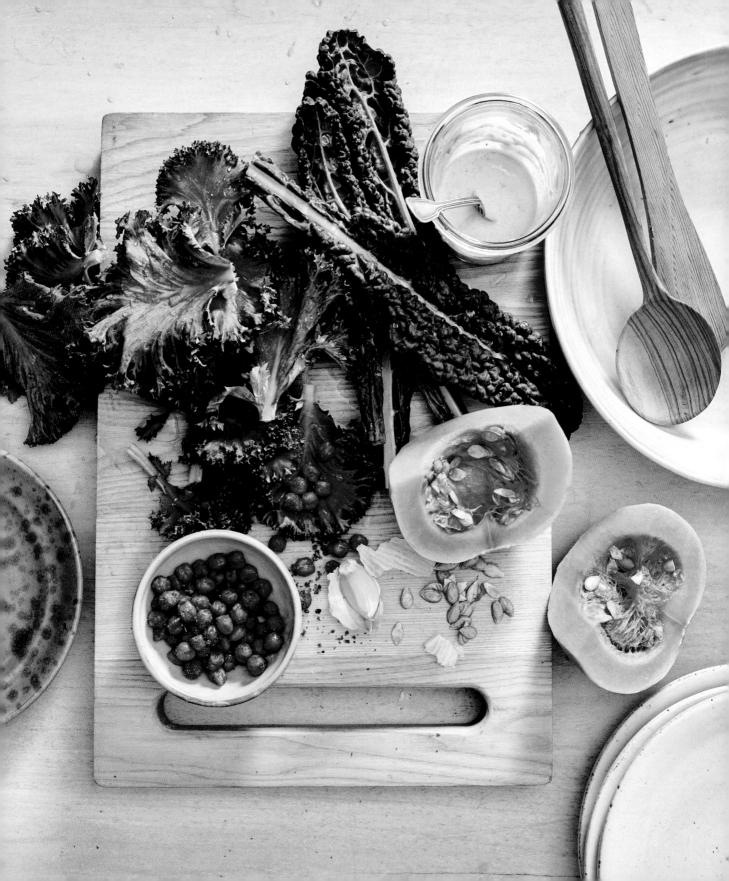

KALE CAESAR!

FOR THE DRESSING

½ cup raw cashews, soaked in boiling water for at least 30 minutes or in room-temperature water overnight

½ teaspoon vegan Worcestershire sauce

½ teaspoon Dijon mustard (preferably whole grain)

1 garlic clove, minced

3 tablespoons nutritional yeast

Juice of 1 lemon

½ to 1 cup water

Salt and freshly ground black pepper, to taste

FOR THE SALAD

1 bunch (about 1 pound) of lacinato kale, tough stems removed

Juice of ½ lemon

Pinch of salt

½ cup canned no salt added chickpeas, rinsed and drained

1 tablespoon capers

3 tablespoons unsalted roasted sunflower seeds

NEURO 9 ITEMS: cashews, kale, chickpeas, sunflower seeds

PREP TIME: 15 minutes, not including the 30 minutes of soaking

COOKING TIME: none

TOTAL TIME: 15 minutes

YIELD: 3 servings

In a blender, blend all dressing ingredients until smooth, adding about ½ cup water or as needed to get the desired consistency; season with salt and pepper to taste.

Shred the kale leaves into bite-size pieces and add to a mixing bowl. Sprinkle with lemon juice and salt. Massage the kale for about 1 minute, or until softened but still crunchy. Alternatively, massage the kale with 1 to 2 tablespoons of the dressing.

Toss kale, chickpeas, and capers in a bowl with 2 to 3 tablespoons of the dressing; divide the salad among three serving bowls. Drizzle with some extra dressing and scatter extra capers and sunflower seeds on top.

Recipe Note

- *Roast the chickpeas with paprika, garlic powder, and cumin for 30 minutes at 350°F for extra crunch.*

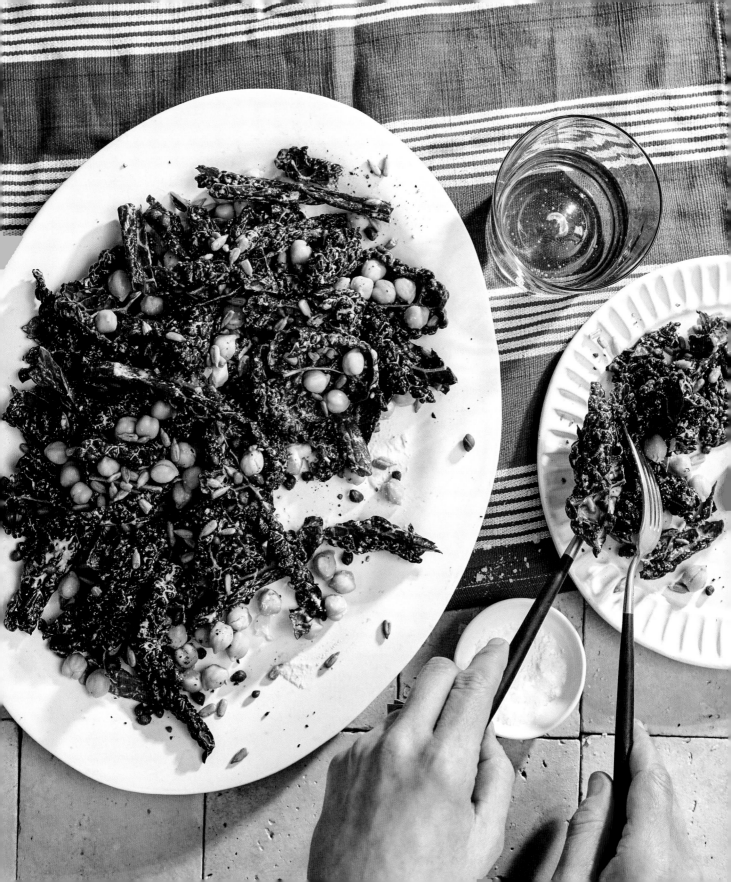

ASIAN CUCUMBER SALAD WITH SPICY GREEN TEA TANGERINE DRESSING

FOR THE DRESSING

1½ teaspoons low-sodium tamari or liquid aminos

Pinch Korean red pepper powder (gochugaru) or red pepper flakes

Juice and zest of 1 tangerine

½ teaspoon matcha green tea powder

1 tablespoon rice vinegar (or to taste)

½ teaspoon finely grated fresh ginger

Salt and freshly ground pepper, to taste

FOR THE SALAD

2 English cucumbers, cut in half, deseeded, and sliced

1 cup mushrooms, sliced

½ cup thinly sliced radishes

3 scallions, thinly sliced

1 fresh red chili, deseeded and finely chopped

¼ cup fresh Thai basil or cilantro, finely chopped

3 tablespoons chopped roasted peanuts or cashews

NEURO 9 ITEMS: herbs and spices, nuts

PREP TIME: 10 minutes

COOKING TIME: none

TOTAL TIME: 10 minutes

YIELD: 3 servings

In a blender, blend together all dressing ingredients and season to taste; set aside.

Add all salad ingredients to a bowl and toss with the dressing. Serve immediately.

Recipe Note

- *For a creamier dressing, add a tablespoon of peanut butter.*

MEXICAN QUINOA CHIPOTLE SALAD

FOR THE DRESSING

Juice of 1 large lime

½ cup Almond Chipotle Sauce (page 209)

Salt and freshly ground pepper, to taste

FOR THE SALAD

1 cup cooked tricolor quinoa

1 15-ounce can no salt added pinto or black beans, rinsed and drained

1 small red onion, chopped

1 red bell pepper, chopped

1 jalapeño pepper, seeds and pith removed, chopped

2 medium tomatoes, deseeded and diced

1½ cups shredded lettuce

½ avocado, pitted and sliced

1 bunch cilantro, leaves only, chopped

½ teaspoon each of garlic powder and cumin

NEURO 9 ITEMS: almonds, quinoa, beans, lettuce, herbs and spices

PREP TIME: 15 minutes

COOKING TIME: none

TOTAL TIME: 15 minutes

YIELD: 3 servings

Whisk together the lime juice with the Almond Chipotle Sauce, add a tablespoon of water to thin, if needed, season with salt and pepper, and set aside.

Mix quinoa, beans, onion, and bell pepper, then add jalapeño, tomatoes, lettuce, avocado, and cilantro. Add the spices and toss with the dressing. Adjust seasoning, if needed, and serve.

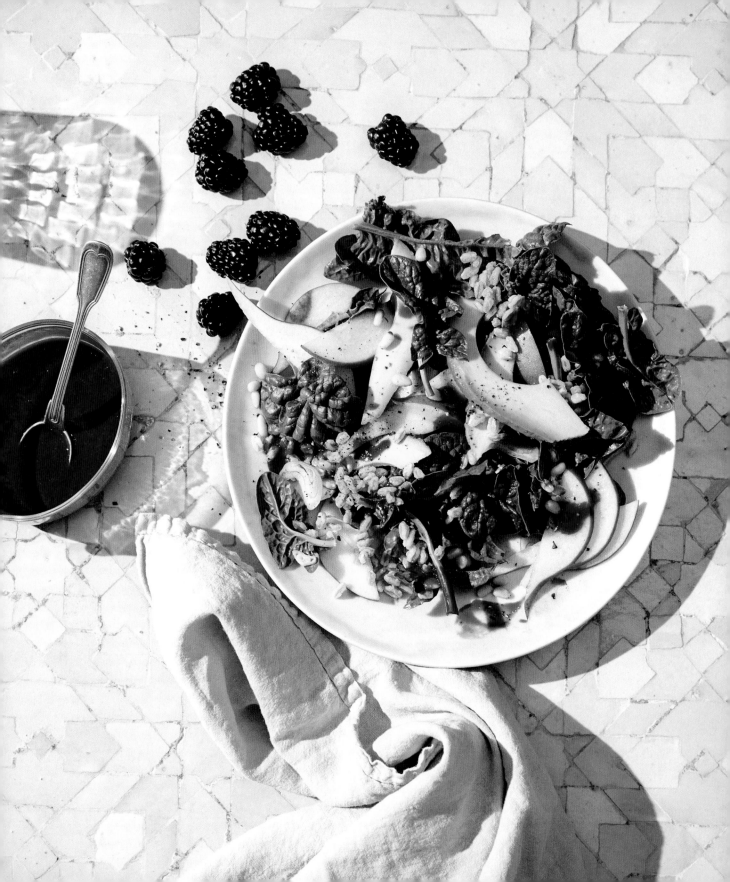

SPINACH FARRO SALAD
WITH BLACKBERRY DRESSING

FOR THE DRESSING

2 tablespoons balsamic vinegar

Juice of 1 lime

2/3 cup fresh or frozen blackberries

1/2 teaspoon fresh ginger, finely grated

Sea salt and freshly ground black pepper, to taste

FOR THE SALAD

6 cups baby spinach

1 cup cooked farro

1/2 medium Bosc pear, cored and thinly sliced

1 avocado, pitted and sliced

1 shallot, thinly sliced

3 tablespoons lightly toasted pine nuts

NEURO 9 ITEMS: spinach, farro, blackberries, pine nuts

PREP TIME: 20 minutes

COOKING TIME: none

TOTAL TIME: 20 minutes

YIELD: 3 servings

Blend together all dressing ingredients in a blender and strain through a fine-meshed sieve; season to taste and set aside.

Combine spinach, farro, pear, avocado, and shallot in a large bowl and toss with the dressing. Scatter the pine nuts on top before serving.

Recipe Notes

- *This is an easily adaptable salad and can be tweaked to suit your taste.*

- *Try using raspberries instead of blackberries in the dressing, and add peach instead of pear.*

- *Substitute the farro with cooked lentils and the pear with shaved fennel.*

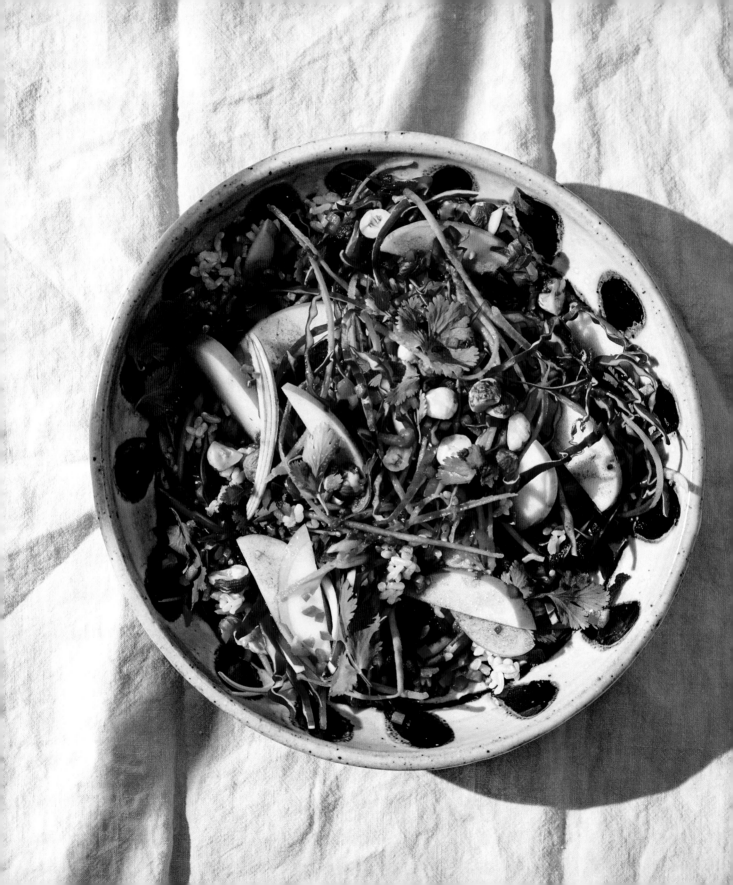

CRUNCHY ZESTY WINTER SALAD

FOR THE DRESSING

⅓ cup fresh red grapefruit juice (or orange juice)

1 teaspoon finely grated fresh ginger

1 red chili pepper, deseeded and finely chopped (or ¼ teaspoon cayenne pepper)

3 tablespoons balsamic vinegar

1 teaspoon whole-grain mustard

2 teaspoons EVOO

Salt and freshly ground black pepper, to taste

FOR THE SALAD

1 cup cooked brown rice

1 apple, cored and thinly sliced

3 cups red cabbage, shredded

1 large carrot, peeled and grated

1 baby beet, peeled and grated

½ red onion, thinly sliced

Handful of fresh cilantro or parsley, chopped

½ cup lightly toasted hazelnuts, chopped

NEURO 9 ITEMS: brown rice, cabbage, herbs, and hazelnuts

PREP TIME: 20 minutes

COOKING TIME: none

TOTAL TIME: 20 minutes

YIELD: 3 servings

Whisk together all dressing ingredients and season to taste; set aside.

Combine brown rice, apple, cabbage, carrot, beet, onion, and cilantro in a large bowl and toss with the dressing. Adjust seasoning, if needed, and scatter the hazelnuts on top before serving.

Recipe Notes

- *Add one segmented small orange to the salad.*

- *Use pears instead of apples.*

BROAD BEAN SUMAC TAHINI SALAD

FOR THE DRESSING

3 tablespoons tahini

½ teaspoon harissa (or hot sauce)

Juice and zest of 1 large lemon

1 teaspoon sumac (or to taste)

2 tablespoons nutritional yeast

1 garlic clove, crushed

Salt and freshly ground black pepper, to taste

FOR THE SALAD

1 cup fresh or frozen broad beans (outer skin discarded)

9 medium spears asparagus, trimmed and cut into 1-inch pieces

⅔ cup fresh peas

2 medium celery stalks, thinly sliced

1 medium carrot, coarsely grated

½ medium red onion, thinly sliced

2 romaine lettuce hearts

Handful of pea shoots or other microgreens (optional)

NEURO 9 ITEMS: tahini, broad beans, lettuce, microgreens, herbs and spices

PREP TIME: 15 minutes

COOKING TIME: 2 minutes

TOTAL TIME: 17 minutes

YIELD: 3 servings

Whisk all dressing ingredients in a bowl until smooth, adding enough water to get the desired consistency; season to taste.

Blanch broad beans, asparagus, and peas in boiling water until just tender, about 2 minutes. Drain and tip into iced water to cool, then drain well and add to a bowl. Add celery, carrot, onion, lettuce, and pea shoots, if using, to the bowl and mix to combine.

Pour dressing over the salad, toss to coat, and serve. Top with some microgreens and sumac.

Recipe Notes

- *You may substitute the broad beans with lima beans.*
- *Add a few artichoke hearts (packed in water) to the salad.*

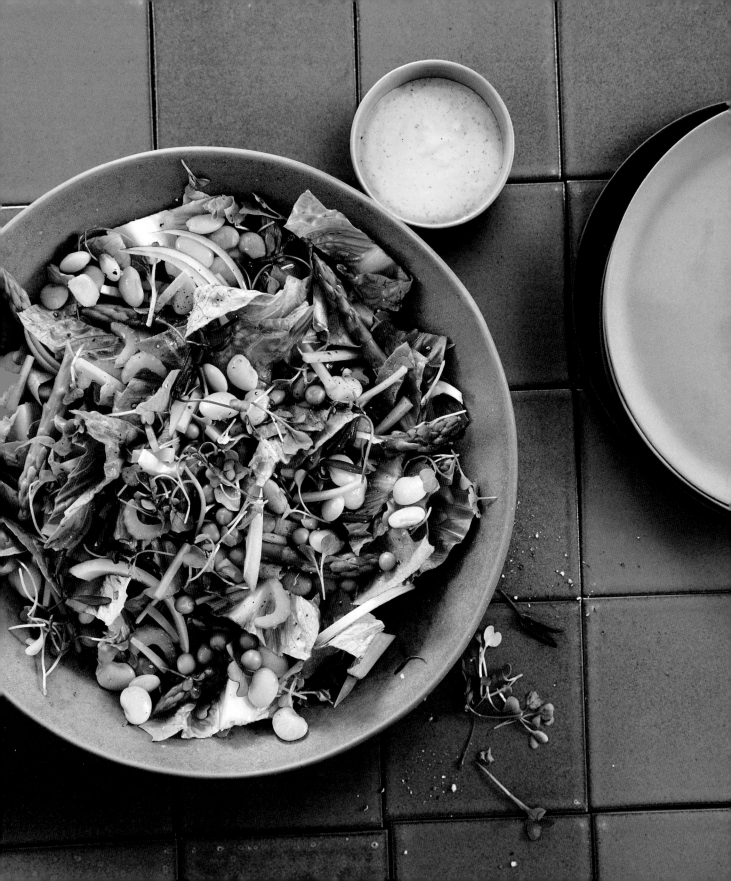

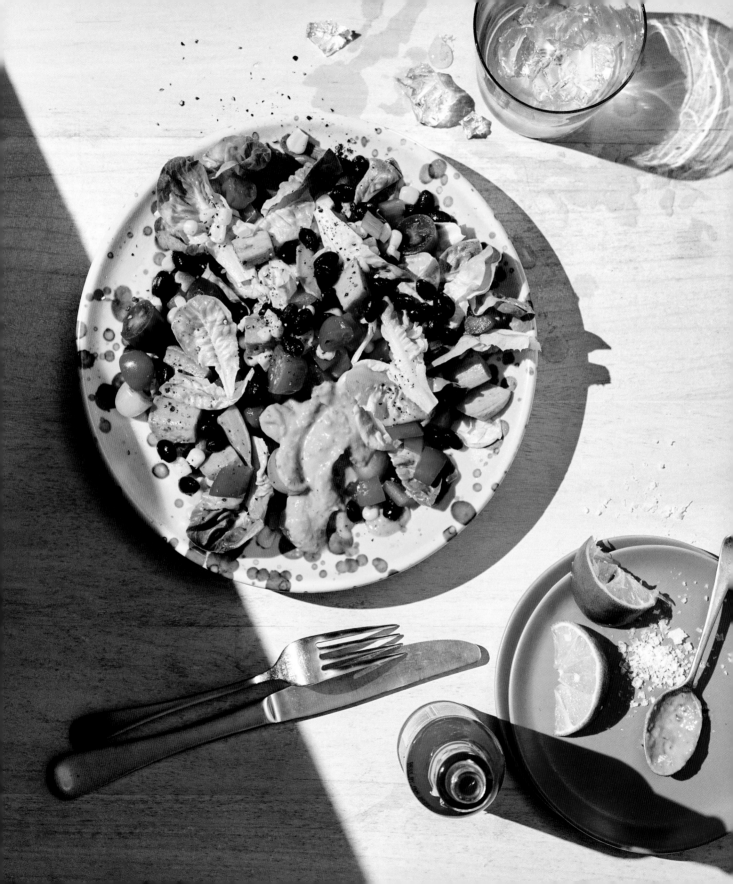

SOUTH OF THE BORDER SALAD

FOR THE DRESSING

1 ripe avocado, pitted and sliced

1 shallot, roughly chopped (or ½ small red onion)

1 teaspoon chipotle powder

1 teaspoon cumin powder

Juice and zest of 1 large lime

2 tablespoons fresh cilantro leaves

1 garlic clove, minced

1 tablespoon apple cider vinegar

½ cup water

Salt and freshly ground black pepper, to taste

FOR THE SALAD

1 medium sweet potato, cooked (boiled, baked, or microwaved) and diced

1 cup corn, thawed if frozen

½ medium bell pepper (any color), deseeded and diced small

1 cup cherry or grape tomatoes, halved

1 cup canned no salt added black beans, drained and rinsed

Bunch of cilantro, chopped

3 cups spring salad mix

¼ cup pumpkin seeds (or sunflower seeds)

NEURO 9 ITEMS: salad greens, beans, pumpkin seeds, herbs and spices

PREP TIME: 15 minutes

COOKING TIME: none

TOTAL TIME: 15 minutes

YIELD: 3 servings

For the dressing, blend all dressing ingredients in a blender until smooth and creamy, adding enough water, if necessary, to get the desired consistency. Season to taste and set aside.

Mix sweet potato, corn, bell pepper, tomatoes, and beans in a bowl; add cilantro and spring salad mix; drizzle with the dressing and toss lightly. Sprinkle with pumpkin seeds and serve.

Recipe Notes

- *Substitute sweet potato with sliced grilled zucchini or grilled asparagus.*
- *Refrigerate the salad and dressing separately for up to two days.*

RAINBOW SALAD WITH TURMERIC DRESSING

FOR THE DRESSING

3 tablespoons each of lemon and orange juice

½ teaspoon each of ground turmeric and cumin

3 tablespoons tahini

½ teaspoon orange blossom water (optional)

Salt and freshly ground black pepper, to taste

FOR THE SALAD

6 medium rainbow carrots cut into thin ribbons with a peeler or spiralized

5 to 6 radishes, thinly sliced

½ English cucumber, thinly sliced

1 head butter lettuce, shredded

1 bunch of watercress, shredded

Handful of fresh mint leaves, shredded

1½ cups cooked chickpeas

NEURO 9 ITEMS: spices (including turmeric), lettuce, watercress, herbs, tahini, chickpeas

PREP TIME: 20 minutes

COOKING TIME: none

TOTAL TIME: 20 minutes

YIELD: 3 servings

Whisk all dressing ingredients until smooth, adding a few tablespoons of water if necessary to get the desired consistency.

Combine carrots, radishes, cucumber, lettuce, watercress, and mint in a salad bowl. Scatter chickpeas on top, drizzle with the dressing, and serve.

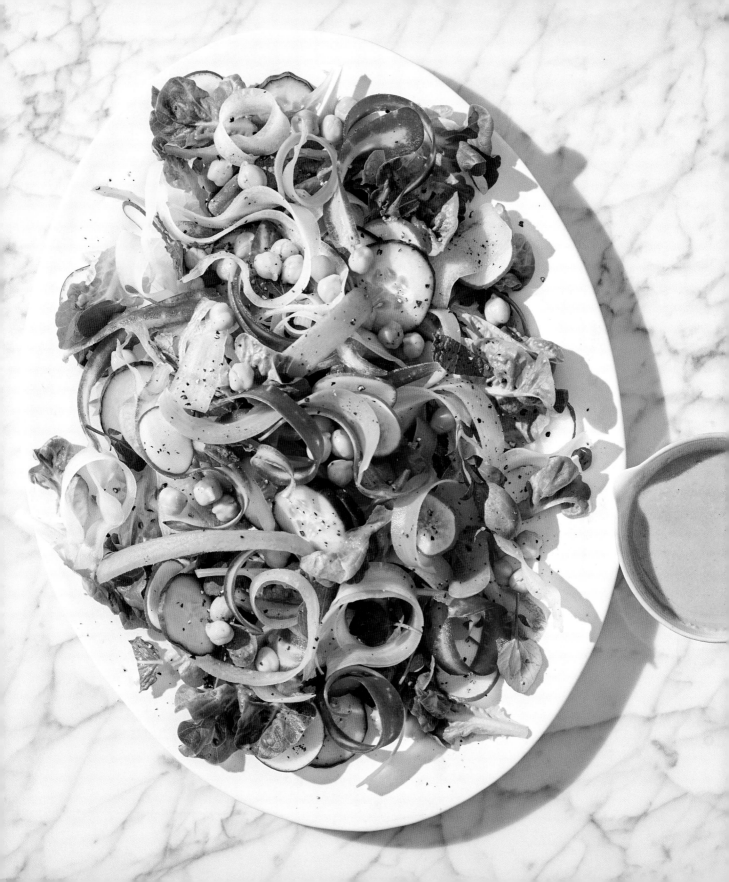

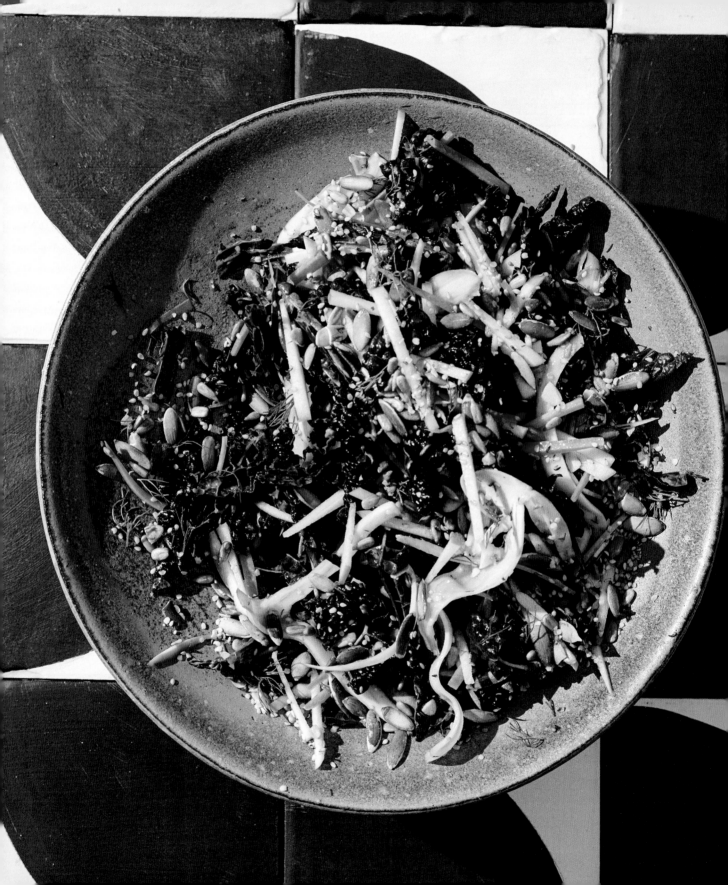

KALE FENNEL SEED SALAD

FOR THE SALAD

1 large bunch (about 1 pound) of kale, tough stalks discarded, sliced into thin ribbons

1 teaspoon each of lemon juice and EVOO

Pinch of salt

2 large carrots, coarsely grated or cut into matchsticks

1 fennel bulb, trimmed and thinly sliced

1 small green apple, peeled and cut into matchsticks

4 tablespoons mixed seeds (e.g., pumpkin, sunflower, hemp, and sesame seeds)

FOR THE DRESSING

Juice of 1 small orange (about ½ cup)

2 tablespoons lime or lemon juice

2 teaspoons Dijon mustard

4 tablespoons finely chopped fennel fronds or dill

Salt and freshly ground black pepper, to taste

NEURO 9 ITEMS: kale, seeds

PREP TIME: 15 minutes

COOKING TIME: none

TOTAL TIME: 15 minutes

YIELD: 3–4 servings

Add the kale to a salad bowl; drizzle with the lemon juice and EVOO and sprinkle with a generous pinch of salt. Gently massage the kale for about 2 minutes, or until it softens.

Add the carrots, fennel, and apple and toss to combine.

Whisk the dressing ingredients in a small bowl and season to taste with salt and pepper; pour over the salad and toss lightly, then sprinkle the mixed seeds on top and serve.

Recipe Notes

- *Add 2 tablespoons tahini to thicken the dressing. You can refrigerate leftover dressing for up to five days.*

- *Add a cup of cooked quinoa, lentils, or roasted vegetables to make this a hearty meal.*

LENTIL AND ROASTED BUTTERNUT SQUASH SALAD

FOR THE VINAIGRETTE

1 tablespoon tahini

½ teaspoon whole-grain Dijon mustard

1 tablespoon balsamic vinegar

2 tablespoons apple cider vinegar

1 shallot, chopped

Salt and freshly ground black pepper, to taste

FOR THE SALAD

1½ cups cooked Puy or green lentils, drained

1½ cups roasted butternut squash, diced

2 cooked golden beets, peeled and sliced

1 small zucchini, cut into very thin strips

2 packed cups mixed baby salad leaves

¼ cup lightly roasted hazelnuts, chopped

NEURO 9 ITEMS: greens, lentils, hazelnuts

PREP TIME: 10 minutes

COOKING TIME: none

TOTAL TIME: 10 minutes

YIELD: 3 servings

In a blender, blend all dressing ingredients until smooth, adding a little water if necessary to get the desired dressing consistency; set aside.

Add lentils, butternut squash, beets, zucchini, and baby greens to a large bowl and mix to combine.

Drizzle salad with dressing and toss lightly; adjust the seasoning to taste and divide salad among three serving bowls. Scatter hazelnuts on top and serve.

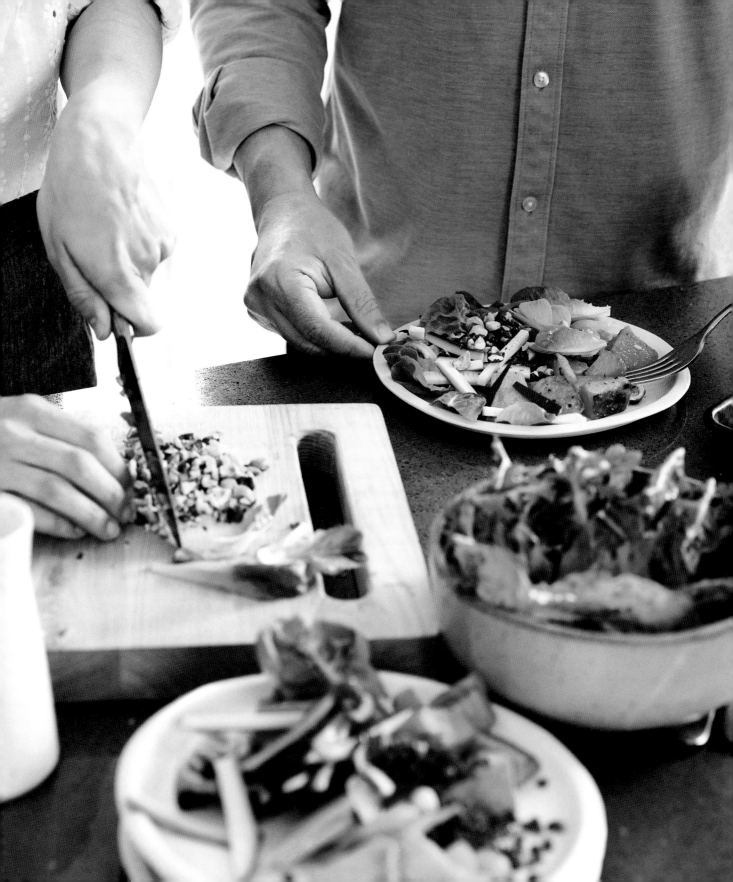

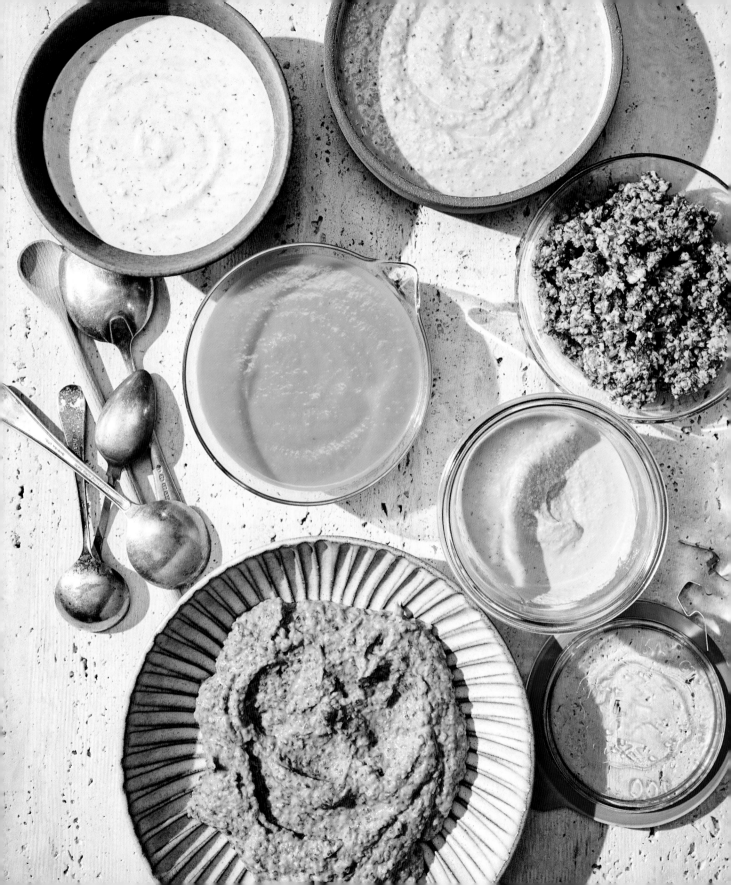

CASHEW SOUR CREAM

1½ cups raw cashews, soaked in boiling water for at least 1 hour or in room-temperature water overnight

¾ cup water

2 tablespoons fresh lemon juice

2 teaspoons apple cider vinegar

¼ teaspoon salt

NEURO 9 ITEMS: cashews

PREP TIME: 5 minutes, not including the 1 hour or more of soaking

COOKING TIME: none

TOTAL TIME: 5 minutes

YIELD: 2 cups

Place cashews in a bowl and cover with boiling water. Soak for at least 1 hour or overnight if you have the time. Rinse and drain. Place the drained cashews in a blender. Add the water, lemon juice, vinegar, and salt. Blend on high until super smooth. Add a little more water to help with blending. Transfer into a glass container. The cream will thicken up as it chills.

CHIPOTLE CASHEW QUESO

1½ cups raw cashews

¼ cup nutritional yeast

½ teaspoon salt

¼ teaspoon garlic powder

½ teaspoon cumin

¼ teaspoon chili powder

1 large or 2 small chipotle peppers in adobo sauce (sold in cans at grocery stores; add more peppers if you can handle the heat!)

1 cup boiling hot water, plus more as needed to make the queso thinner

NEURO 9 ITEMS: cashews, cumin

PREP TIME: 10 minutes

COOKING TIME: none

TOTAL TIME: 10 minutes

YIELD: 8 servings

Add the cashews, nutritional yeast, spices, and chipotle peppers to a high-speed blender (such as a Vitamix). Blend on high, scraping the sides down intermittently, to make a spread. Add small amounts of hot water through the top opening while the blender is running, and slowly blend the ingredients into a thick, spreadable cheese consistency. Serve over salads, burritos, nachos, or with vegetables as a dip.

SPICY GREEN HUMMUS

1 15-ounce can no salt added chickpeas, drained and rinsed

2 garlic cloves

¼ cup tahini

2 cups cilantro leaves and stems, chopped (or parsley or dill)

1 small jalapeño, seeds and pith removed (leave the seeds if you want extra kick to it)

Juice of 1 large lemon

Salt, to taste

NEURO 9 ITEMS: chickpeas, tahini, herbs

PREP TIME: 15 minutes

COOKING TIME: none

TOTAL TIME: 15 minutes

YIELD: 6 servings

In a food processor, place the chickpeas, garlic cloves, and tahini and blend until creamy and smooth. Add the cilantro, jalapeño, and lemon juice; blend until smooth. Add some water if the hummus is quite thick. Taste and adjust heat with more jalapeño, garlic for a "zing," or acid with more lemon. Add a pinch of salt if needed. Serve as a dip or as a spread on wraps and sandwiches.

PESTO BEAN DIP

2 15-ounce cans cannellini beans, drained and rinsed

2 cups basil leaves

¼ cup nutritional yeast

3 tablespoons tahini

Juice of 2 large lemons

3 garlic cloves

¼ teaspoon salt

Pinch of cayenne pepper (optional)

Freshly ground black pepper, to taste

NEURO 9 ITEMS: cannellini beans, tahini, herbs and spices

PREP TIME: 5 minutes

COOKING TIME: none

TOTAL TIME: 5 minutes

YIELD: 16 servings

Blend all ingredients in a blender. Add more lemon juice, cayenne pepper, and garlic to taste.

CASHEW RANCH DRESSING

1 cup raw cashews

½ cup unsweetened almond milk

1 tablespoon lemon juice

1 garlic clove, peeled

½ teaspoon salt

¼ teaspoon black pepper

¼ teaspoon onion powder

1 teaspoon apple cider vinegar

1 tablespoon nutritional yeast

¼ cup chopped fresh dill

NEURO 9 ITEMS: cashews, herbs

PREP TIME: 5 minutes, not including the 30 minutes of soaking

COOKING TIME: none

TOTAL TIME: 5 minutes

YIELD: 8 servings

Soak the cashews in boiling water for at least 30 minutes, or in room-temperature water overnight to soften. While cashews are soaking, measure out almond milk and add lemon juice; set aside to curdle.

Drain and rinse cashews. Transfer them to a powerful blender and add the almond milk and lemon juice mixture, garlic, salt, pepper, onion powder, vinegar, and nutritional yeast. Blend on high for 1 to 2 minutes or until very creamy and smooth. Then add half of the dill and pulse several times to incorporate (you don't want it fully puréed).

Taste and adjust flavor as needed, adding more salt, lemon juice, or vinegar for acidity, garlic for garlic flavor, or herbs for a more herbal flavor. Chop the rest of the dill finely and mix it in the dressing (don't blend it). This dressing will thicken in the refrigerator.

ROASTED CARROT DRESSING

4 medium-size carrots, chopped into 1-inch pieces

Avocado oil spray

¼ teaspoon ground cumin

¼ cup white wine vinegar

¼ cup water

Juice and pulp of 1 large orange

¼ teaspoon salt

NEURO 9 ITEMS: spices

PREP TIME: 10 minutes

COOKING TIME: 40 minutes

TOTAL TIME: 50 minutes

YIELD: 16 servings

Preheat the oven to 375°F. Line a baking sheet with a silicone baking mat or parchment paper and place the carrots in a single layer; spray with avocado oil. Roast for 30 to 40 minutes until tender.

Add the carrots and the rest of the ingredients to a blender or food processor and blend until smooth.

Let cool completely before using to allow the flavors to mix.

GREEN CHUTNEY

1 large bunch of cilantro leaves with tender stems (about 2 cups)

1 bunch of mint leaves, stems removed (about 1 cup)

1 cup walnuts

1 large serrano or jalapeño pepper with seeds, pith, and stem removed

Juice of 2 large lemons

2 to 3 garlic cloves, peeled

¼ teaspoon salt, adjust to taste

½ cup water

NEURO 9 ITEMS: herbs, walnuts

PREP TIME: 10 minutes

COOKING TIME: none

TOTAL TIME: 10 minutes

YIELD: 6 servings

Place all the ingredients in a food processor and pulse until smooth, scraping the sides a few times. Don't overblend to make a "smoothie"; a little texture is better.

ALMOND CHIPOTLE SAUCE

1 cup water

½ cup raw almonds

1 chipotle pepper in adobo sauce (from a jar or a can)

2 tablespoons lime or lemon juice

3 tablespoons nutritional yeast

2 cloves garlic

Salt and pepper to taste

NEURO 9 ITEMS: almonds

PREP TIME: 5 minutes

COOKING TIME: none

TOTAL TIME: 5 minutes

YIELD: 6-8 servings

Blend all ingredients and serve. Keep in the refrigerator for 5 days to a week.

CHIA BERRY JAM

NEURO 9 ITEMS: berries, chia seeds

PREP TIME: 3 minutes

COOKING TIME: 5–7 minutes

TOTAL TIME: 8–10 minutes

YIELD: 20 servings

2 cups fresh or frozen mixed berries

1½ tablespoons freshly squeezed lemon juice

3 tablespoons monk fruit sweetener (or to taste)

2½ tablespoons chia seeds

Combine berries, lemon juice, sweetener, and chia seeds in a large saucepan and heat over medium-low heat. Reduce the heat to low and cook, stirring occasionally, for about 5 to 7 minutes, or until the berries soften and release their juices.

If you prefer a smoother consistency, mash the berries with a potato masher or blend with an immersion blender. Transfer the jam to a jar or other airtight glass container.

Allow the jam to set for at least 15 minutes before serving. Refrigerate for up to five days or freeze for up to two months.

Recipe Note

- **NO-COOK JAM:** *Combine all ingredients in a large bowl, adding an extra ½ tablespoon chia seeds if necessary. Mash or blend to get the desired consistency and allow to set for 5 to 10 minutes before serving. Refrigerate for up to three days or freeze for up to one month.*

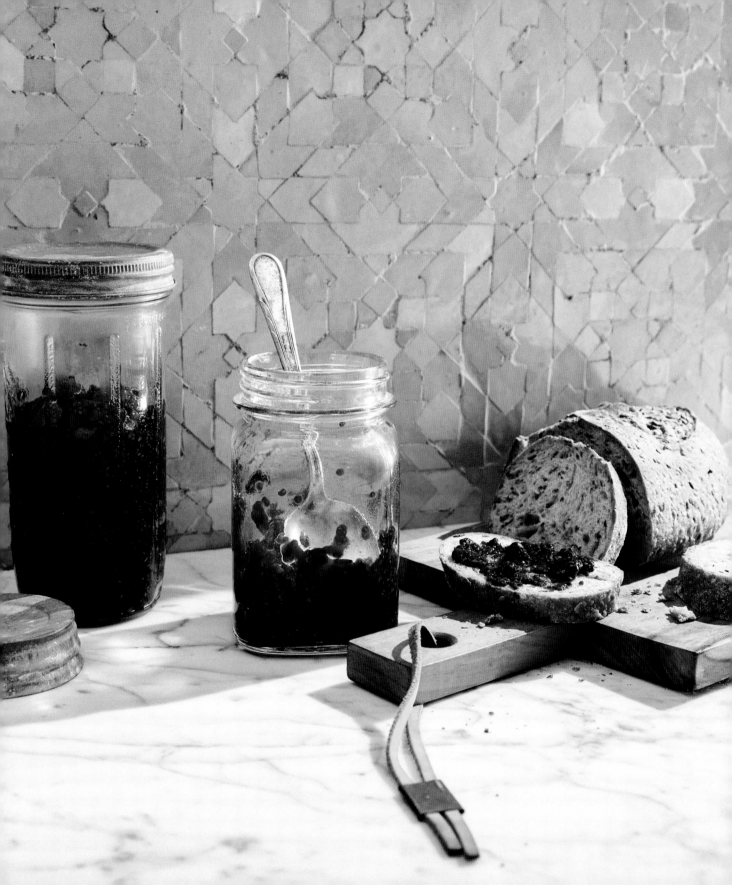

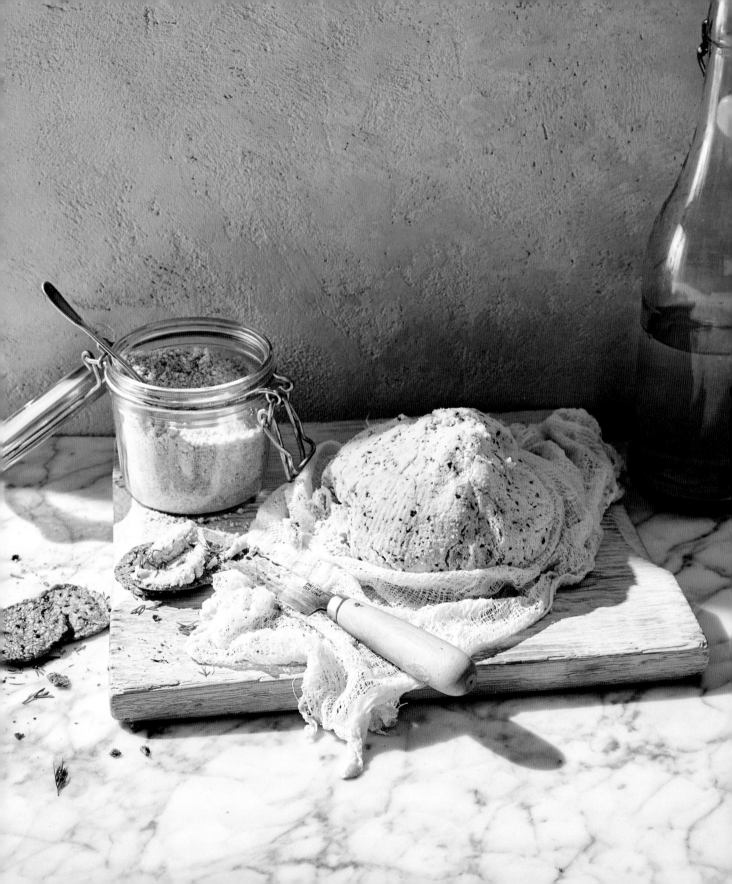

FERMENTED CASHEW CHEESE WITH HERBS

NEURO 9 ITEMS: cashews, herbs

PREP TIME: 30 minutes, not including the 30 minutes of soaking

FERMENTATION AND REFRIGERATION TIME: 12 hours

COOKING TIME: none

TOTAL PREPARATION TIME: 30 minutes

YIELD: 12 servings

2 cups raw cashews

1 garlic clove, minced

2 tablespoons lemon juice

3 tablespoons nutritional yeast

½ teaspoon garlic powder

½ teaspoon salt

½ cup water

2 probiotic capsules (with at least 50 billion CFU, or colony forming units)

TOPPINGS

2 tablespoons finely minced fresh dill

Freshly ground colorful pepper (red, white, and black peppercorns)

OR

1 teaspoon smoked paprika, 1 teaspoon dried oregano, 1 teaspoon nutritional yeast, 1 tablespoon finely chopped walnuts, and a pinch of salt

Place cashews in a bowl and cover with cool water. Soak the cashews in boiling water for 30 minutes, or overnight in room temperature water to soften. Once soaked, drain cashews thoroughly and add to a food processor or blender. Add minced garlic, lemon juice, nutritional yeast, garlic powder, and salt and process until very creamy and smooth, scraping down the sides as needed. Add the water a little at a time until a creamy consistency is reached. Taste and adjust seasonings as needed, adding more lemon juice for acidity, nutritional yeast for cheesiness, and garlic for zing.

Transfer mixture to a mixing bowl. Break the probiotic capsules and add the "powder" into the mixture. Stir with a wooden spoon to combine well.

Place a colander or a fine mesh strainer over another mixing bowl. Layer it with one or two layers of cheesecloth (or a kitchen towel). Spoon the cashew cheese mixture over the cheesecloth. Then gather the corners and gently twist the top to form the cheese into a "disc." Secure with a twisty or a rubber band.

Leave to set on the countertop at room temperature for at least 48 hours. Leave it for another 24 hours to get a tangier taste. Then refrigerate for at least 12 hours to firm. Once it's chilled, unwrap very gently and coat with dill, or spices. If parts of it fall off, re-form by pressing it firmly back into the disc. Place back in the fridge to harden.

The cheese will be ready to consume in 3 to 4 days. Serve chilled with seed crackers, vegetables, and fruits.

CASHEW PARMESAN

1 cup raw cashews

4 tablespoons nutritional yeast

½ teaspoon salt

½ teaspoon garlic powder

2 tablespoons sesame seeds (optional)

NEURO 9 ITEMS: cashews, sesame seeds

PREP TIME: 5 minutes

COOKING TIME: none

TOTAL TIME: 5 minutes

YIELD: 16 servings

Add all ingredients to a food processor and mix/pulse until a fine meal is achieved. Stores for two months in an airtight container in the refrigerator.

ALMOND SOFT CHEESE

NEURO 9 ITEMS: almonds, herbs

PREP TIME: 5 minutes

COOKING TIME: none

REFRIGERATION TIME: 2 hours

TOTAL TIME: 2 hours and 5 minutes

YIELD: 12 servings

2 cups slivered blanched almonds

2 to 3 teaspoons nutritional yeast, plus more to taste

2 tablespoons lemon juice

½ teaspoon sea salt

Dash of garlic powder

¾ cup water

2–3 tablespoons finely chopped fresh basil, oregano, or parsley (optional)

Add almonds, nutritional yeast, lemon juice, salt, garlic powder, and water to a high-speed blender and blend until smooth and creamy, scraping down the sides as needed (about 2 minutes). You want a puréed mixture with no bits of almonds intact. Add a bit more water a little at a time if the mixture is having a hard time blending until smooth.

Taste and adjust flavor as needed, adding more salt for overall flavor, nutritional yeast for cheesiness, and lemon juice for acidity. For more flavor, add some fresh basil, oregano, or parsley.

If the mixture is too thin and "watery," spread cheesecloth in a colander and scoop over the cheesecloth. Then gather the corners and gently twist the top to form the cheese into a ball. Secure with a rubber band and place into a fine mesh strainer set over a mixing bowl for 1 to 2 hours. This will allow the "cheese" to firm up a bit.

Unwrap carefully and transfer to a glass bowl with a tight lid. Place in the fridge to make firm. The cheese will be ready to consume in 2 hours. To serve, spread on toast or use as stuffing in lasagnas or stuffed pasta shells.

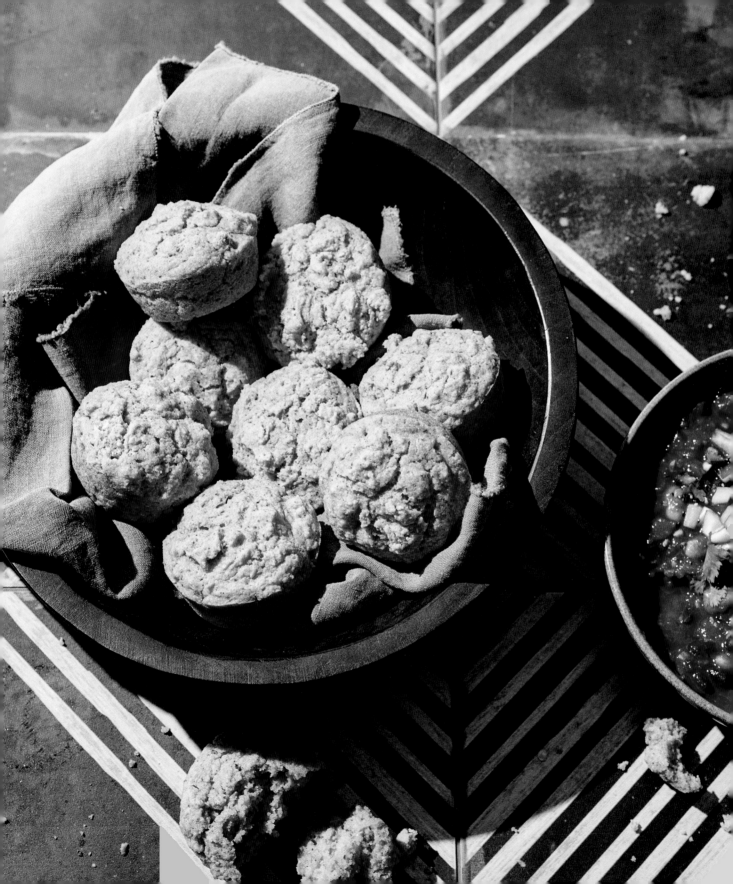

CORNBREAD MUFFINS

NEURO 9 ITEMS: flaxseeds, 100% whole-wheat flour, (whole) cornmeal

PREP TIME: 10 minutes

COOKING TIME: 25 minutes

TOTAL TIME: 40 minutes

YIELD: 12 servings

1 tablespoon flax meal plus 3 tablespoons water

2 teaspoons apple cider vinegar

1 cup soy milk

1 cup 100% whole-wheat flour

1 cup fine ground cornmeal

3 teaspoons baking powder

Pinch of salt

2 tablespoons applesauce

1 tablespoon EVOO

Preheat the oven to 350°F. Lightly spray a 12-cup muffin pan with cooking spray or line with parchment paper cups.

In a small bowl, make the flax "egg" by mixing the flax meal and water. Set aside.

In a separate bowl, add the vinegar to the milk and let curdle for 5 minutes.

In a large bowl, mix together the flour, cornmeal, baking powder, and salt. Add the soy milk, flax "egg," applesauce, and EVOO. Use a wooden spoon to fold the dry and wet ingredients together. Don't overmix.

Spoon the batter into the muffin cups and bake for 20 to 25 minutes until muffin edges are golden brown. Remove from the oven and let cool for about 10 minutes, then transfer muffins to a cooling rack. Serve, preferably warm and with chili!

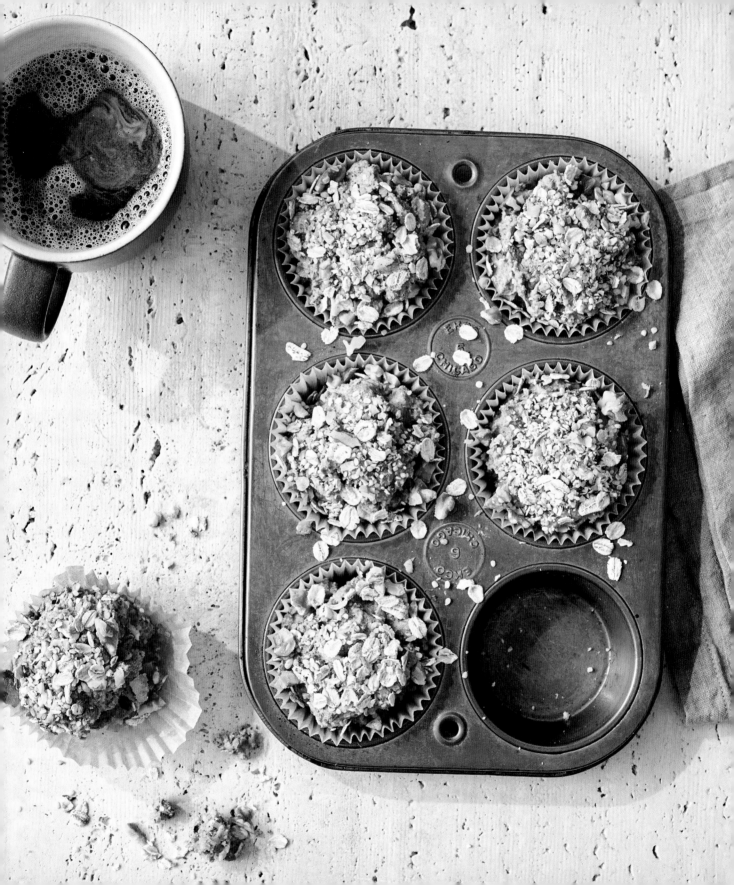

OMEGA MUFFINS

NEURO 9 ITEMS: oats, hemp seeds, flaxseeds, walnuts, tahini, cinnamon (spice)

PREP TIME: 10 minutes

COOKING TIME: 25 minutes

TOTAL TIME: 35 minutes

YIELD: 8 muffins

2 cups oat flour

½ cup plus 2 tablespoons rolled oats

1½ teaspoons baking powder

3 tablespoons hemp seeds, divided

3 tablespoons ground flaxseeds

1 teaspoon baking soda

½ teaspoon ground cinnamon

Pinch of salt

⅔ cup plus 2 tablespoons chopped walnuts

1 small Granny Smith apple, peeled, cored, and grated

⅓ cup ripe banana, mashed

2 teaspoons apple cider vinegar

3 tablespoons EVOO

1¼ cups unsweetened plant-based milk, preferably soy (more as needed)

Preheat the oven to 400°F. Line 8 cups of a muffin tin with paper cups and set aside.

Mix oat flour, ½ cup rolled oats, baking powder, 2 tablespoons hemp seeds, ground flaxseeds, baking soda, cinnamon, and salt in a large bowl. Lightly stir in ⅔ cup walnuts and grated apple until coated with the mixture.

Whisk banana, apple cider vinegar, EVOO, and soy milk in another bowl and pour into the dry ingredients, stirring until incorporated. Do not overmix. If the batter is too thick, add a little milk.

Divide the batter into the prepared muffin cups; sprinkle with the remaining rolled oats, hemp seeds, and walnuts. Bake for about 25 minutes, or until golden. Transfer the muffins to a wire rack and let cool to room temperature before serving.

The muffins will keep in an airtight container refrigerated for up to three days and frozen for up to a month.

Recipe Note

- *Substitute EVOO with nut butter of choice.*

SPELT BLUEBERRY SCONES

NEURO 9 ITEMS: blueberries

PREP TIME: 10 minutes

COOKING TIME: 15 minutes

TOTAL TIME: 25 minutes

YIELD: 8 scones

⅔ cup unsweetened plant-based milk, preferably soy, plus 2 tablespoons for glazing

2 teaspoons lemon juice

2½ cups spelt flour

1½ teaspoons baking powder

4 tablespoons monk fruit sweetener

Zest of 1 small lemon

1 cup fresh blueberries

3 tablespoons EVOO, or applesauce for oil-free version

⅓ cup applesauce

¼ teaspoon each of sea salt and ground cinnamon

Preheat the oven to 375°F and line a baking sheet with parchment paper or a silicone baking mat; set aside.

Mix milk with the lemon juice and set aside for a few minutes to sour.

Mix flour, baking powder, monk fruit sweetener, and lemon zest in a large mixing bowl, then add the blueberries and toss lightly until they are coated in the mixture. Add EVOO, applesauce, and the soured milk.

Mix lightly, using a spatula, until the mixture comes together, adding a little more milk or flour as needed to form a soft, sticky dough. Do not overmix.

Transfer the dough onto a lightly floured work surface and pat into an about 1-inch-thick circle. Cut into eight triangles and transfer to the baking sheet.

Brush the scones with a little plant-based milk and bake for 12 to 15 minutes, or until golden. Let the scones cool before serving.

Recipe Note

- *Serve with some almond butter and Chia Berry Jam (page 210)*

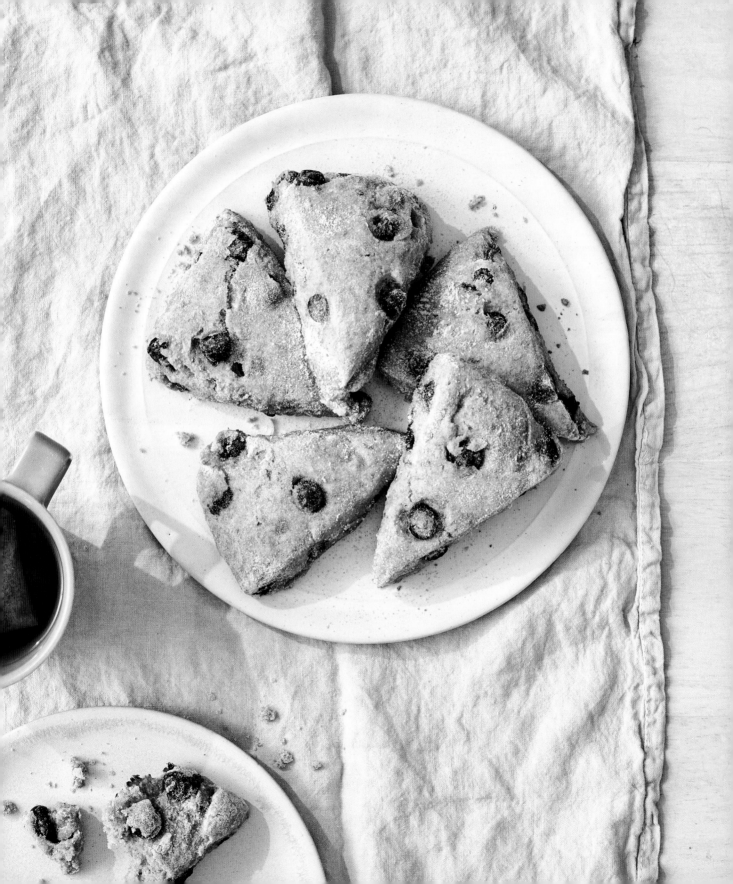

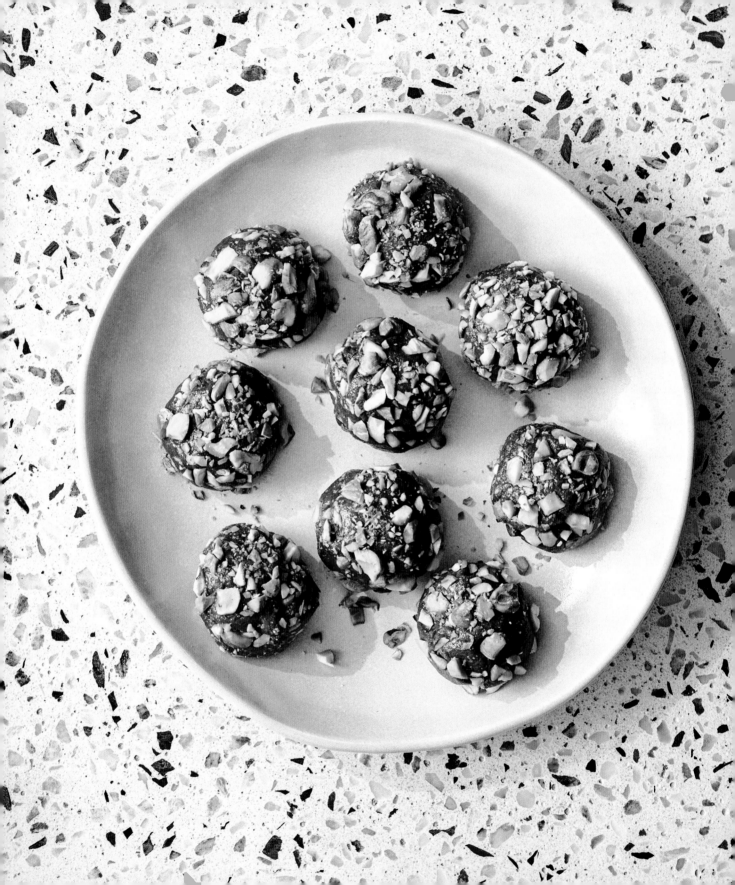

DARK CHOCOLATE ORANGE PISTACHIO TRUFFLES

NEURO 9 ITEMS: almonds, other nuts, flaxseeds

PREP TIME: 10 minutes plus 30 minutes of freezing

COOKING TIME: none

TOTAL TIME: 40 minutes

YIELD: 16 truffles

⅓ cup sugar- and dairy-free dark chocolate or chocolate chips

1 cup almond flour (more as needed)

3 tablespoons monk fruit sweetener (optional)

2 tablespoons raw cacao powder

2 tablespoons ground golden flaxseeds

Pinch of salt

Juice and zest of 1 large orange

½ cup almond butter

⅓ cup toasted unsalted pistachios, chopped

Line a small baking sheet with parchment paper and set aside.

To create a double boiler to melt the chocolate chips, take a large saucepan, place it over medium-high heat, and add 2 inches of water and bring to a boil. Then place a medium glass or ceramic mixing bowl on top of the saucepan, making sure it is not touching the water in the saucepan. Place the chocolate in the bowl and let it melt, stirring frequently with a spatula to evenly distribute the heat and help it melt faster. Once the chocolate is melted, remove from heat.

Combine almond flour, monk fruit, cacao powder, flaxseeds, salt, and orange zest in a mixing bowl. Add the almond butter and melted chocolate and stir until smooth. Adjust the consistency, if needed, with extra almond flour if too soft and runny or with a little orange juice if too dry and hard. You want it to feel like cookie batter, sticky enough to form into a ball.

Scooping the mixture with a teaspoon, form into small balls. Roll in chopped pistachios and place in the freezer for about 30 minutes to firm up before serving.

Store in an airtight container in the refrigerator for up to a week or in the freezer for up to a month.

PEANUT BUTTER TAHINI ENERGY BITES

1 cup unsalted peanut butter

¼ cup tahini

½ cup plus 2 tablespoons oat flour (more, if needed)

2 heaped tablespoons raw hemp seeds

½ teaspoon cinnamon (or to taste)

2 tablespoons monk fruit (or to taste)

A generous pinch of salt

GARNISHES

Sesame seeds, cacao nibs, chopped dates, and chopped nuts

NEURO 9 ITEMS: tahini, peanuts, oat flour, hemp seeds, other seeds, cinnamon (spice)

PREP TIME: 10 minutes plus 15 minutes of freezer time

COOKING TIME: none

TOTAL TIME: 10 minutes

YIELD: 18 bites

Line a small baking sheet with parchment paper and set aside.

Add all ingredients to a bowl and stir until well-combined.

Using a tablespoon measuring spoon, scoop the mixture and form it into balls. Roll into the desired garnishes and arrange on the prepared baking sheet and let firm up in the freezer for about 10 to 15 minutes.

Transfer the bites to an airtight container and keep refrigerated for up to a week or freeze for up to a month.

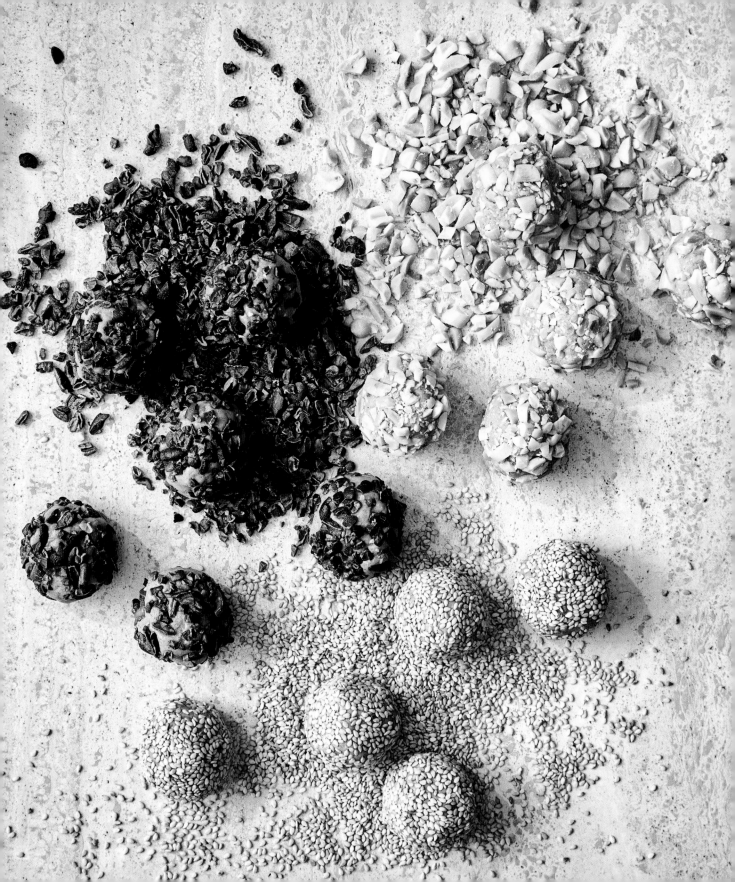

CHOCOLATE HAZELNUT CRUST WITH BERRIES

NEURO 9 ITEMS: hazelnuts, pistachios, berries

PREP TIME: 30 minutes

COOKING TIME: 10 minutes

TOTAL TIME: 40 minutes

YIELD: 16 servings

3 cups roasted unsalted hazelnuts

8 large medjool dates, pitted (9 if they are small)

3 tablespoons cacao powder or unsweetened cocoa powder

Pinch of sea salt

FOR THE COCO-HAZELNUT BUTTER

3 cups roasted unsalted hazelnuts

4 tablespoons cacao powder or unsweetened cocoa powder

3 tablespoons monk fruit sweetener (more to taste)

1 teaspoon pure vanilla extract

¼ teaspoon sea salt

TOPPINGS

Raspberries, blueberries, strawberries, blackberries, pistachios (crushed), and mint leaves

Place raw hazelnuts in a food processor or high-speed blender. Pulse until they are processed into a meal. Place the meal in a dish and set aside.

Place the dates in the food processor and process until small bits form a ball. Stop the processor and add the cacao or cocoa, salt, and half of the hazelnut meal. Pulse until mixed together. Continue adding the hazelnut meal little by little until the dough gets more formed and sticks together.

Once you have a dough, line an 8-by-8-inch (for a thicker crust) or 11-by-7-inch (for a thinner crust) baking dish with parchment paper and press the mixture into the dish to make an even layer. Place in the refrigerator or freezer to harden into a crust.

FOR THE COCO-HAZELNUT BUTTER: Preheat the oven to 350°F and add hazelnuts to a baking sheet in a single layer. Roast for 8 to 10 minutes just to warm the natural oils and loosen the skins. If raw, roast for a total of 12 to 15 minutes. This will make it easier to blend into butter.

Remove hazelnuts from the oven and cool slightly. Then transfer to a large kitchen towel and use your hands to roll the nuts around and remove most of the skins. You want to get as much as possible off for a creamier butter.

Leaving excess skin behind, add hazelnuts to a high-speed blender. Blend on low until a butter is formed, about 8 to 10 minutes total, scraping down the sides as needed.

Once the hazelnut butter is creamy and smooth, add the cacao or cocoa powder, monk fruit sweetener, vanilla, and salt and blend well. Taste and adjust seasonings as needed, adding more vanilla if desired.

TO ARRANGE: Take the hazelnut crust out of the refrigerator or freezer and roughly spread 2 to 3 tablespoons of the coco-hazelnut butter over the crust (the goal is to make the fruit stick to the crust). Arrange the berries in any pattern you like. Drizzle 2 to 3 tablespoons of the butter on top of the fruit (you may need to warm it up slightly to make it drizzle at this point). Sprinkle crushed pistachios on top and place mint leaves around. Serve by slicing squares diagonally.

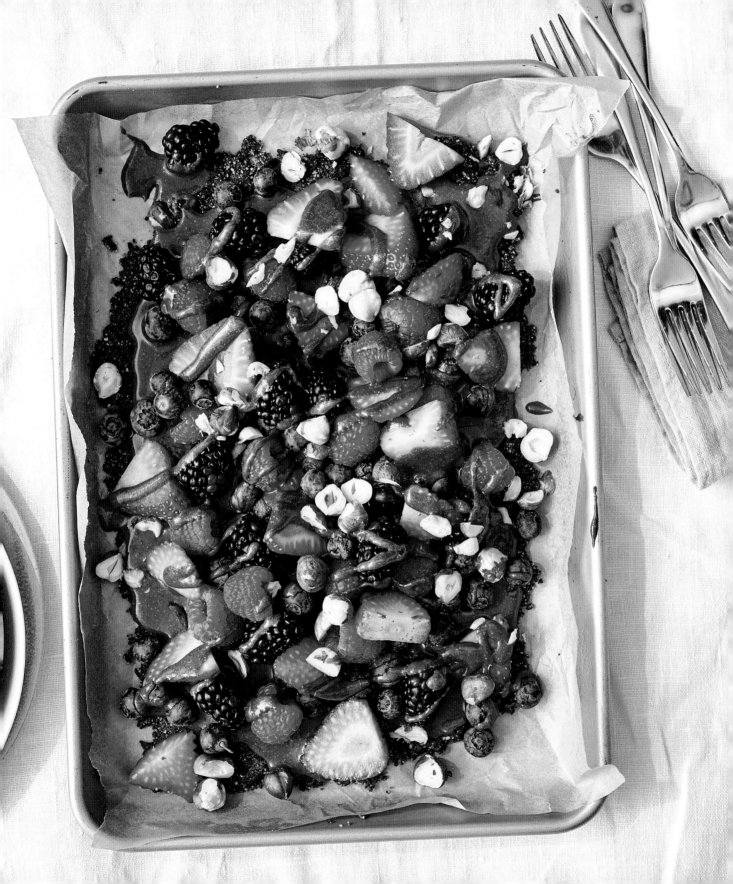

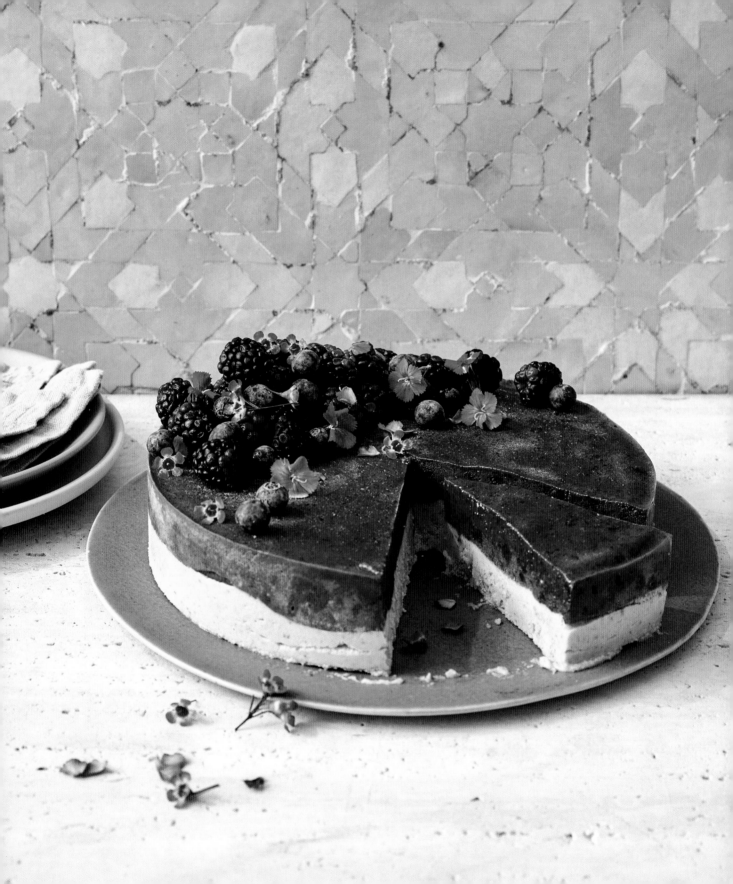

BERRY NICE CREAM CAKE

FOR THE VANILLA NICE CREAM CAKE LAYER

2 cups raw cashews, soaked in water for 4 hours or, better, overnight

2 very ripe bananas with brown spots, sliced into 1-inch-thick slices, arranged on a plate and frozen for 4 hours or overnight

1 cup pitted medjool dates (about 10 dates)

Seeds from ½ vanilla pod (or ½ teaspoon vanilla extract)

¼ cup unsweetened soy milk as needed to thin the nice cream

FOR THE BERRY LAYER

2 cups frozen blueberries

1 cup soy milk, and more to thin as needed

½ cup dates

1 cup raw walnuts

NEURO 9 ITEMS: cashews, walnuts, blueberries

PREP TIME: 15 minutes plus 8 hours of freezing time

COOKING TIME: none

TOTAL TIME: 8–9 hours

YIELD: 12 servings

Soak the cashews and freeze the banana slices either overnight or at least 4 hours before starting.

In a blender, blend soaked cashews, frozen bananas, dates, and vanilla together until smooth and creamy, adding as little soy milk as possible. Spread into a pan. Place in the freezer for at least 2 hours.

FOR THE BERRY LAYER: In a blender, blend blueberries, soy milk, dates, and walnuts until smooth. Carefully spread over the top of the vanilla nice cream cake layer and put in the freezer for 2 to 3 hours or until set.

Dip a large knife in hot water and cut the cake; serve with fresh berries, nuts, flowers, or fresh herbs. Let it soften a little before eating so it's creamier.

Recipe Note

- *You can drizzle some coco-hazelnut butter on top of the cake (Chocolate Hazelnut Crust with Berries, page 226).*

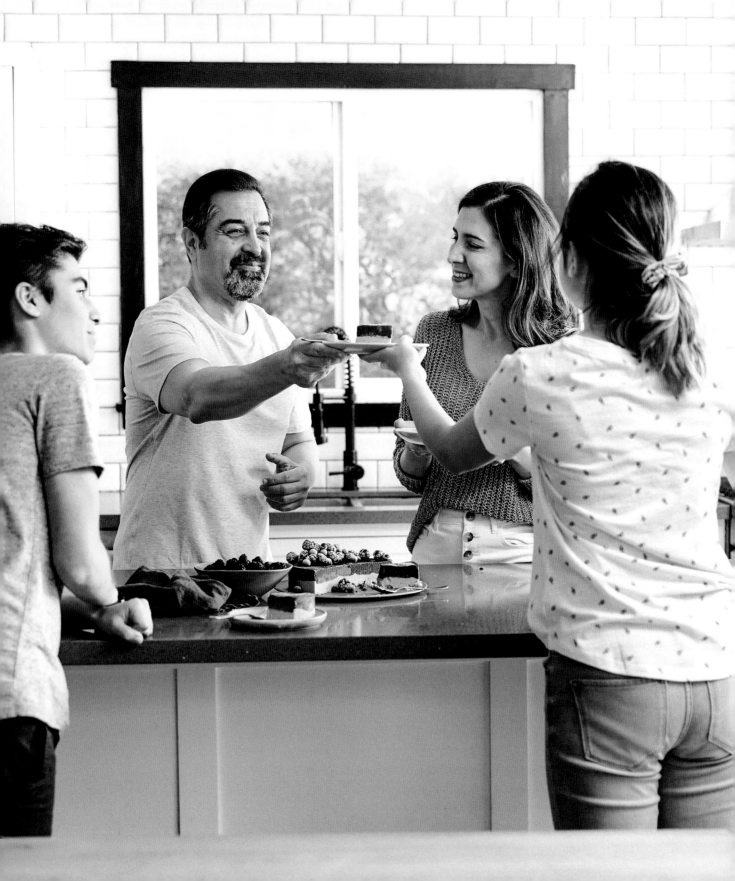

AFTERWORD

Science and medicine change with new information. We learn more about diseases like Alzheimer's every day, and we may in fact see a pharmacological treatment sometime in the near future. But why wait for that moment, and why continue living a life that will force you to someday rely on medication? Lifestyle change is available right now, and as you've seen throughout this book, our patients have transformed their lives using simple, effective, personalized techniques, and it's entirely within your power to do the same!

Personalized medicine, a model of medical care that customizes treatment based on individual differences in genes, proteins, and environment, has emerged as the new medical paradigm for chronic disease. There's tremendous amount of funding for studies that use this approach, and many medical specialists and scientists are trying to frame their research so that it fits some version of personalized medicine.

The idea behind personalized medicine is that though humans are on the whole very similar, we are very different at the molecular level. Each of us has different metabolic processes and responds to environmental stimuli differently; we process nutrients, minerals, and medications differently. Conventional medicine's approach has been to treat us as though we're all the same, to assume somehow that one nutrient, drug, or behavioral change model fits all. One study says that a vitamin is good for you and we all decide to take it. A drug is found to decrease blood pressure and we're all given prescriptions. We now know that our individual differences profoundly impact the way medical treatments affect us, and also how effective they are. To date, personalized medicine has been used most successfully in the treatment of diabetes, obesity, and heart disease, where doctors look at the unique genetic and molecular constituents of an individual's disease, and, more important, implement lifestyle changes that take into consideration the individual's history, resources, limitations, and proclivities. This comprehensive approach is bringing to light what we discovered years ago: chronic disease, especially neurodegenerative disease, is highly complex and highly personal, and if individuals, families, and communities are given the appropriate resources they can change their own and their family's health better than any hospital, clinic, or academic institution.

The protocol we shared with you in *The 30-Day Alzheimer's Solution* is personalized medicine for the brain. We know this disease is more than just about amyloid and tau, and its cure is certainly not going to be found in a one-size-fits-all approach. Alzheimer's is a multidimensional disease that at its core has glucose and lipid dysregulation, inflammation, oxidation, and degenerative aspects that are in turn affected by individual nutrient deficiencies and toxicities, as well as immune, endocrine, and metabolic factors. We also know that Alzheimer's, and for that matter most diseases of cognition, are deeply affected by the risks you accumulate throughout life and that any lifestyle protocol designed to minimize these risks must take your unique situation into account. Each of these factors needs to be addressed at the level of the individual: and the complex diseases of the brain require personalization at every step.

Bringing about lasting change in people's lives also demands this level of personalization. Compliance with medication varies, as does compliance with lifestyle changes, all based on our individual strengths and weaknesses, and the habits we've created over our lifetimes. Accounting for all these elements is the only way to fight complex chronic diseases of the brain and manifest the full power of our amazing minds.

We believe this book, which we humbly refer to as a "Life Plan," is the future of health. Within these pages, you can find the tools to get control over your brain health and truly experience your optimal life. More than just another diet, protocol, or health book, what you gain by reading these pages and using the carefully designed tools are the means to change your life.

The next step is for you to bring this powerful approach into your life, your family's life, and beyond—into schools, faith communities, businesses, and the larger community. We're doing everything we can to spread this message through our social media community (Sherzai MD), and our nonprofit, Healthy Minds Initiative, to reach communities throughout the world. Please join us in sharing this life plan and sparking a prevention-based revolution.

ACKNOWLEDGMENTS

The reality is that our healthcare system is designed to care for people who are in the full grip of a disease, rather than preventing the onset. As such, millions of families and communities have suffered and will continue to suffer from mostly preventable chronic diseases such as dementia and stroke. This book is, first and foremost, an acknowledgment of their courage and resilience in the face of tremendous challenges and difficulties.

We also dedicate this book to the memory of our grandfathers, whose life in the world of public health and education shaped who we are as physicians and citizens. Both of these remarkable men faced many battles, but none greater than the battle they fought to the very end of life. Witnessing their courageous fight with dementia was what brought the two of us together and ultimately led us to our focus on preventive neurology and public health at the community level. In every patient we've seen in our clinics, in every attempt to understand the origins and causes of this devastating disease, we remember the struggles of these two great men. They inspired us to write this book, which we hope will make a difference in the lives of many other grandfathers, grandmothers, fathers, and mothers.

We thank the many mentors who taught us the art of research and clinical practice, and the wonderful patients and communities in Loma Linda and San Bernardino who have allowed us to pursue our passion for prevention and have made the experience less like a job and more a joyous journey of discovery.

We are grateful for our friendship with Douglas Abrams, our agent and a dear friend. His kindness and wisdom in every conversation has helped us not only bring our books to life but has made us better humans in the process.

We would like to thank the talented team at HarperOne, especially our editors, Sydney

Rogers and Gideon Weil, for their steadfast support and their empowering leadership that allowed us to stay true to our vision. A special thanks to Colin Price and his creative team for bringing our recipes to life with his gift of food photography.

Our great appreciation to Nikki Van De Carr, whose amazing ability to hear our voices, see our experiences, and help us tell our story was second to none.

We are incredibly grateful to our mothers for their unmitigated love and support on this amazing journey. We would also like to thank our amazing children and partners, Alex and Sophie (also known as "The Science Kids"), who endured many nights of writing, whiteboard sessions, and passionate discussions while listening patiently and sharing their thoughts. And finally, we would like to thank our team and community of the Beach Cities Health District who have partnered with us in our community-based effort to revolutionize the world of brain health through our nonprofit, Healthy Minds Initiative (www.HealthyMindsInitiative.org).

NOTES

1. "Major Depression among Adults," National Institute of Mental Health, nimh.nih.gov/health/statistics/prevalence/major-depression-among-adults.shtml.

2. Martha Clare Morris et al., "MIND Diet Associated with Reduced Incidence of Alzheimer's Disease," *Alzheimer's & Dementia* 11.9 (2015) 1007–14.

3. Yue Ruan et al., "Dietary Fat Intake and Risk of Alzheimer's Disease and Dementia: A Meta-Analysis of Cohort Studies," *Current Alzheimer Research* 15.9 (2018): 869–76; Smita Eknath Desale et al., "Role of Dietary Fatty Acids in Microglial Polarization in Alzheimer's Disease," *Journal of Neuroinflammation* 17.1 (2020): 1–14; Ryu Takechi et al., "Dietary Fats, Cerebrovasculature Integrity and Alzheimer's Disease Risk," *Progress in Lipid Research* 49.2 (2010): 159–70.

4. O. I. Okereke et al., "Dietary Fat Types and 4-Year Cognitive Change in Community-Dwelling Older Women," *Annals of Neurology* 72, no. 1 (2012): 124–34.

5. Anya Topiwala et al., "Moderate Alcohol Consumption as Risk Factor for Adverse Brain Outcomes and Cognitive Decline: Longitudinal Cohort Study," *BMJ* 357 (2017): j2353.

6. C. K. Maki et al., "A Meta-Analysis of Randomized Controlled Trials that Compare the Lipid Effects of Beef versus Poultry and/or Fish Consumption," *Journal of Clinical Lipidology* 6, no. 4 (2012): 352–61.

7. F. Jernerén et al., "Brain Atrophy in Cognitively Impaired Elderly: The Importance of Long-Chain Ω-3 Fatty Acids and B Vitamin Status in a Randomized Controlled Trial," *The American Journal of Clinical Nutrition* 102, no. 1 (2015): 215–21.

8. Roy M. Pitkin et al., "Dietary Reference Intakes for Thiamin, Riboflavin, Niacin, Vitamin B6, Folate, Vitamin B12, Pantothenic Acid, Biotin and Choline," National Academy Press (Washington, DC: 2000).

9. Emma Derbyshire, "Could We Be Overlooking a Potential Choline Crisis in the United Kingdom?" *BMJ Nutrition, Prevention & Health* (2019).

10. Alina Solomon et al., "Midlife Serum Cholesterol and Increased Risk of Alzheimer's and Vascular Dementia Three Decades Later," *Dementia and Geriatric Cognitive Disorders* 28.1 (2009): 75–80.

11. J. George Fodor et al., "'Fishing' for the Origins of the 'Eskimos and Heart Disease' Story: Facts or Wishful Thinking?" *Canadian Journal of Cardiology* 30.8 (2014): 864–68; Marie-Ludivine Chateau-Degat et al., "Cardiovascular Burden and Related Risk Factors among Nunavik (Quebec) Inuit: Insights from Baseline Findings in the Circumpolar Inuit Health in Transition Cohort Study," *Canadian Journal of Cardiology* 26.6 (2010): e190–e196.

12. Geng Zong et al., "Whole Grain Intake and Mortality from All Causes, Cardiovascular Disease, and Cancer:

A Meta-Analysis of Prospective Cohort Studies," *Circulation* 133.24 (2016): 2370–80.

[13] Sandro Altamura and Martina U. Muckenthaler, "Iron Toxicity in Diseases of Aging: Alzheimer's Disease, Parkinson's Disease and Atherosclerosis," *Journal of Alzheimer's Disease* 16.4 (2009): 879–95.

[14] Ayesha Z. Sherzai et al., "Mediterranean Diet and Incidence of Stroke in the California Teachers Study," *Circulation* 131.1 (2015): AMP85.

INDEX